BEYOND SYMPTOMS

How to Create an Extraordinary Life Using the Knowledge, Tools, and Rituals of the ULTRA HEALTHY

Dr. Cotey Jordan

Writing & Publishing Process by PlugAndPlayPublishing.com
Book Cover by Tracey Miller | TraceOfStyle.com
Edited by Jenny Butterfield

ISBN-13: 978-1724397799
ISBN-10: 1724397796

Disclaimer: This book contains opinions, ideas, experiences, and exercises. Please consult your doctor before implementing any strategies or ideas. The purchaser and/or reader of these materials assumes all responsibility for the use of this information. Dr. Cotey Jordan and Publisher assume no responsibility and/or liability whatsoever for any purchaser and/or reader of these materials.

To learn more about Dr. Cotey or have him speak at your event please visit WellnessSpeakerUSA.com.

Dedication

This book is written on behalf of all the men and women who are aware and have embodied the gift we have been given as humans. This is my attempt to reach out to the less fortunate who have not yet been exposed to the life-changing principle of health from within.

This book is dedicated to mankind. This is about you. May this truth bring you hope, inspiration, and empower you to experience extraordinary health for as long as you shall live.

Acknowledgement

The completion of this undertaking could not have been possible without the contribution and support of countless people whose names may not all be enumerated. Their participation is sincerely appreciated and gratefully acknowledged. I would like to, however, express my deep appreciation and indebtedness to a particular and select few:

Amanda - my strong, courageous, and beautiful wife - for your love through the good and bad times. You've supported me in this journey in more ways than I could possibly communicate. Thank You!

You are my Queen. I am your Rock. Together, we will continue to change lives!

Ali and Alex – my young, yet extremely wise and stunning daughters - you both keep me humble, make me laugh, and remind me what life is really about. You are unique individuals and the most phenomenal children a dad could have. I love you both very much.

Dawn Jordan - my mother - for teaching me to be independent, for your amazing quiet strength and wisdom, and for always being so proud of me. Thank you!

Bob Jordan - my dad - for always being a source of support and encouragement. Whether it be coaching me through sports, celebrating my military career or supporting my business ideas, you have never wavered. Thank you!

Bill & Cheryl Albaugh - my In-Laws – for being so willing to jump in over the past few years and help Amanda and I when we needed it most. Thank you!

Table of Contents

Preface

I was inspired to write this book after joining a Men's Group and getting to know one gentleman. After only a few short months, I had witnessed this man create and achieve several goals all while embracing overwhelm and facing life's battles head-on. He had complete control of his life in every aspect imaginable, except one.

This man was sharp, confident and, appeared to be fearless. He was and is successful as the CEO of a family-fun park that had been established for over twenty years. He devoted himself to God, had a supportive and beautiful wife, and together they raised four solid and respectful kids. After getting our families together and spending a Friday night at his home, it became obvious to me why he was unable to fulfill his health goals.

Chris had good intentions. He talked about wanting to be healthy. He said all the right things; "I'd like to change my body and lose some weight;" "I would like to eat clean and workout regularly;" "I'd like to make my health a top priority." But intentions will only take you so far. Even if he truly meant everything he said, the reality is he didn't know what he needed to do. He simply didn't have enough information or direction to be able to follow through.

My wife, Amanda, and I talked early the next morning about the wonderful time we spent with Chris and his family. In the back of my mind, I was itching to reach out to Chris about his health goals. I wanted to help him understand why and how someone so put together, a go-getter, a make-it-happen type person such as himself was unable to achieve the status of health he was seeking. Determined, I told Amanda, "I'm going to write a book that will empower individuals to become super healthy by offering the specific details and directions needed to achieve their health goals." I brainstormed an outline on paper, began typing on my laptop, and by Sunday evening, the main system for extraordinary health that I use regularly was written down in black and white. I spent the next few months filling in the details.

Forgive me in advance for my system's simplicity. My intentions are to change lives with this book – not simply give a rehash of everything you have already been told. Our flawed medical system relies on useless studies, over-complicated procedures, and our health system routinely fails to take into consideration the quality-of-life of the patient. This book is different. The reality of my health is the lifestyle that I've created, which has allowed my family and I to reach and surpass our health goals, is very simple. And that is why this system will work for you too.

I want to help you achieve your goals and become healthy, super healthy even. If you believe that you deserve to be healthier (have more energy, be more productive, look and feel better than you have during your entire life) then this book is for you. Your family, friends, and loved ones deserve the best version of you – so let's give it to them.

-Dr. Cotey Jordan

Destined to Be Healthy

There is an urgent problem facing our country where families are being compromised due to misinformation about health. Americans have never been as sick, diseased, or symptomatic as we are today. There are endless people who are suffering, who have been through the ringer and have tried anything and everything to no avail. For those of you who are suffering from a health condition and your quality of life is nowhere near where you would like it to be, I assure you there is a better way. Health doesn't have to be so complicated. There are answers to all your unanswered questions. There is hope. I know because I have personally used the information in this book to overcome health challenges of my own and regain my youth and vitality. Currently, the lifestyle that I have created and choose to live is leading me towards my destiny and allowing me to fulfill my life purpose.

However, my lifestyle wasn't always like this.

Growing up, my family was misled by the medical system, and I too was put through the ringer. What I remember most about my childhood was always being sick. I would regularly miss school and extracurricular activities. I felt different than the other kids. By the age of ten, I had been experiencing persistent sore throats, an extremely weak immune system, and debilitating migraines. I recall the 2:00 a.m. trips to the ER quite vividly. Reaching for the medicine cabinet and taking pills, which ever medications I could find, and locking myself in a pitch-black room became the norm for me. While most kids were outside and playing with friends, I would cry myself to sleep in the middle of the day just wishing the migraines away. As if this wasn't bad enough, I was still wetting the bed well into my teenage years. You could imagine what that does to a teenage boy's self-esteem. I felt embarrassed. I felt shame and insecure. I felt alone.

Looking back, I needed a way to gain some confidence in my life, so I became a competitive marathoner and I joined the military. While my body appeared to be in peak, physical condition on the outside, I was deteriorating, falling apart, and suffering on the inside. The physical pounding of long-distance running and the long days of military training led my condition to progressively worsen.

The Day My Life Changed

In 2005, when I was gearing up for a twelve-month deployment in support of Operation Iraqi Freedom, the intensity and frequency of my migraines became so severe that they were impacting my quality of life, and I was unable to fully participate in the required military training. Feeling weak and defeated, I found myself in the office of a highly-decorated, Air Force officer who, up until that moment, I had only seen on posters around the Air Force base. I was feeling extremely intimidated, overwhelmed, and even a bit pathetic. I was shocked to find out that I was not being released from duty, sent home, or even punished; instead, this man was reaching out to help me. He insisted that I go to his doctor for my condition. I was confused, hesitant, and absolutely blown away that someone so high up cared about someone like me, who seemed to be so small.

What was even more astounding is not only did this man insist that I see his doctor, he personally drove me to the office that very day. As it turned out, his doctor was a Wellness expert, a specific, subluxation-based Chiropractor.

With no previous experience with chiropractic, I had no idea what to expect or how a chiropractor could potentially help me. I had never experienced an environment nor a doctor like this one. This doctor's office wasn't the standard hurry-up-and-wait, label-me-and-give-me-pills, and send-me-home-defeated office that I had become accustomed to. Instead, the doctor seemed rather curious and interested in getting to understand my condition and how my migraines were affecting my life. He thoroughly examined me in a manner I've never experienced before and took the time to educate me, helping me by making sense of my condition. He explained very clearly why my body was functioning the way it was, then inspired me to take my health into my own hands. I no longer had to rely on medications, injections, or the routine recommendations of the multiple medical doctors who never seemed to have a satisfying answer or effective solution to any of my conditions. I was empowered. I felt in control for the first time in my life, and finally having that power felt amazing!

I went on to serve my year-long deployment in support of Operation Iraqi Freedom - not fully understanding how my life would be forever changed. Some people spend a lifetime seeking out their purpose in this crazy world that we live in, and for whatever reason, in 2005 at the young age of 21, my life's purpose found me.

Now that I'm in my mid 30's, I'm in the best health of my life. I am confident in my body. I feel phenomenal! I'm focused, my energy levels are through the roof, and I'm more productive now than I have ever been in my entire life. And my extraordinary health is all because this one person, a gentleman I didn't even know, went out of his way, took time to reach out to me, and shared a life-changing principle that I had never been exposed to. Not only has he given me my life back, he's made it so that my children will never have to suffer the way I did. For his time and knowledge, I am eternally grateful. Every child, every parent, and every single person deserves to hear this message!

There are millions of people out there who are just like me: people who are suffering and who would do anything and everything for even the slightest bit of hope. This message is for you. If you allow it, the information in this book will transform your life. What I have to tell you will empower you to take control of your health and the health of your loved ones just as I have. Let's get to work.

PART 1

The Journey Beyond Symptoms

1

Healthcare in America: Our System is Broken

"Health is not an occasional act, it is a permanent lifestyle."
Dr. Cotey Jordan

Healthcare in America is confusing, expensive, and extremely overwhelming. I have spent the past twelve years, studying in eleven countries, searching for keys to helping sick people get well and healthy people stronger. What I've observed is that most doctors are hardly ever on the same page when it comes to figuring out the causes of sickness and disease.

The majority of doctors in our healthcare system are wonderful people with good intentions; they want to help people who are suffering and keep their patients well. Unfortunately, these fantastic doctors are working in an incredibly flawed system which limits what they can do for their patients. Our healthcare here in America is run by the pharmaceutical industry who "advise" our doctors what medications to give their patients as well as insurance companies who know next to nothing about health, dictating what procedures and type of care patients are allowed to receive.

The definition of "doctor" is "teacher," and today, our doctors are no longer afforded the time needed to be able to teach their patients about their health conditions or how to live a healthy lifestyle and avoid health issues altogether. I have made the commitment to teach and inspire people to live life to the fullest by empowering them to take their health into their own hands and giving them the information they need to live a healthy lifestyle.

The goal of this chapter is to create a pivot point for you. I want to challenge your thinking because the best way to get people to do something better is to challenge them. Unfortunately, we tend to only focus on our health when we have already lost it. If we can create a pivot point now and shift your current mindset to get you thinking from a proactive standpoint rather than a reactive standpoint, you're going to truly see the long-term benefits of making your health and the health of your family a top priority.

You've Been Lied To

The healthcare system in America is based on the premise that poor health is determined by bad germs, bad luck, or bad genes. The constant fear of symptoms and disease has us trapped in a reactive healthcare system that is failing us. Look around, and you will see signs of this fear everywhere.

We have all been taught and trained to base our health on how we look and how we feel. The problem with this mindset is that it sends us down a rabbit hole chasing symptoms and not addressing the actual issue at hand. While our medical system is merely treating symptoms and attempting to make you feel better, the underlying problem progressively worsens, leading to major health conditions and even disease.

Our approach to healthcare has led to a major predicament; most Americans do not think about their health until they look or feel bad. Unfortunately, the top three killers in America – properly prescribed medications, cancer, and heart disease – are the causes of death we don't see or feel until it's too late.

It's true. Heart disease is the third leading cause of health-related deaths in America. But did you know that the most frequent symptoms of someone who suffers from heart disease is either a heart attack or a stroke? Think about that. Someone can literally feel fine and look fine for years, and out of the blue one day, he or she suffers a massive heart attack or stroke. I can assure you that neither of these conditions develops overnight. In fact, it takes years upon years for the human body to break down enough to be able to experience either of these serious conditions.

The second leading cause of health-related deaths is cancer. There are literally hundreds of different forms of known cancer, yet we have all been taught to think that cancer is cancer. We simply lump all forms of cancer together, and we seek this magical, scientific cure for this dreadful disease we know as cancer. After collecting, raising, and spending trillions of dollars on cancer research, we have nothing to show for this effort, and we remain oh-so-close to "The Cure." If we spent even a fraction of the funds that we spend on cancer research simply educating the masses of what cancer really is and how it develops in the body, people would be empowered to take action to prevent cancer from happening altogether, rather than hoping they don't have bad luck or bad genetics that is going to lead to them having cancer.

Lastly, the number one health condition that Americans are dying from year after year is properly prescribed medications. The key words there are "properly prescribed," meaning patients are taking their medications exactly as they are instructed. Sadly, this statistic doesn't even include addictions, overdoses, or the fact that most Americans have several doctors, none of which are aware of each other and all of which are prescribing different medications that are not recommended to be prescribed with other meds. And let's not overlook that we're all quite aware that every single medication on the market has side -effects, most of which are worse than the symptom the original drug is being consumed for in the first place. Then of course when the side-effects kick in, we need to take another medication to help with that symptom as well. It's a vicious cycle. We have a huge drug problem in our country, and for whatever reason, nobody is questioning this cycle or prescribing madness.

QUIZ TIME

Whenever I present at workshops, seminars, or in front of large groups, I like to put together mini quizzes to get my audience engaged and creatively thinking for themselves. These questions are not meant to stump anyone, rather they are meant to get people thinking from a different perspective. When you step back and remove yourself completely (past experiences, opinions, and emotions), what is happening with healthcare in our country becomes obvious.

1. Which country in the world spends the most amount of money on its healthcare?

At the time of this writing, National Health Expenditures highlights that "the United States is spending over ***two trillion dollars a year*** on its healthcare" – and that number is on the rise. To be clear, that's trillion with a "T" and a whole bunch of zero's after it! To give you an idea how significant that number is, the second country on that list spends less than one trillion per year. That means our country spends over twice as much as any other country in the world - about 16% of our gross domestic product – on health care.

2. What country takes the most medications?

At the time of this book being written, Americans make up only 5% of the world population yet we consume over 50% of medications worldwide. There is a time and a place for medications, but this is clearly a drug problem. We have lost all focus on healthcare and have turned into a pill-mill, offering up false hope and quick fixes.

3. Where does America rank in the list of healthiest countries in the world?

When ranking the top forty most developed countries in the world on "being healthy," the World Health Organization (WHO) ranked America as low as #37. Keep in mind that America spends BY FAR the most amount of money on its healthcare, consumes BY FAR more medications than any other country, and still we rank all the way down at the bottom of the poll. I would have to imagine that this does not sit well with a country that strives to be number one in everything that we do.

4. Are Americans healthy?

This is a subjective question, and I'll leave it up to you to decide. Overall, I believe that most people would agree that no, we are not healthy. The reality is we are in a health crisis: five out of every six people in America will die from either cancer or heart disease. Will you be the lucky one?

5. Are you as healthy as you would like to be?

Take a minute to really think about this question. Answer it honestly. It's okay to be vulnerable and shake your head "no." In fact, you may even get a little emotional and uneasy with your reality. I believe that everything happens for a reason, and there is a reason why you're reading this book. Quite frankly I'm excited for you. Your life will never be the same after you finish reading this book!

Your Wake-up Call

The current model is failing…

According to the World Health Organization, over 780,000 Americans are killed each year by conventional medicine and FDA approved prescription drugs. We have grown into a culture where there is a pill for every symptom and inconvenience. We have a massive problem where we abuse medications.

Selling sickness is exactly what happens in today's culture. The medical model and pharmaceutical industry have directly and indirectly anchored people to their diseases and conditions, meaning when these people are told that their health could be different, they don't believe they could get better. They simply don't want to believe it. Their diagnoses and conditions have become their identities. This is a dangerous place to be. Once someone has accepted his diagnosis or condition as his identity – who he or she truly is – helping him see the truth is very difficult. Many who have embraced this new (false) belief will even lash out at the people and professionals who believe that person can be helped.

These false beliefs are one of the reasons why this book will be such a liberation for you. You will have the ability to speak life into people and remind them that they are not weak and defective or bound to break down. Let them know that their bodies are intelligent and strong and able to overcome. Sure, plenty will still believe more in their condition and the drugs to treat it over the greatest intelligence that exists within. But do try to help them anyway. You can only help the people who want to be helped. And you owe it to your loved ones to fight for them.

Application Exercise #1

The next time you're out and about with friends, family, co-workers, or at any one of your organizations, take the opportunity to awaken the people around you! Get everyone's attention, and ask them to participate. Have everyone raise one of their hands up in the air (make it fun, no need to be so serious!) to see that everyone is able and willing to participate. Next, ask them the almighty question, **"With a show of hands, who here has known someone personally, someone close to you, who has suffered from either a heart attack, stroke, or cancer?"** Have them keep their hands up, and look around the room. It doesn't matter if there's five people, thirty people, or hundreds of people... the results are always the same. There WILL be a mass majority (> 90%) of hands that go up, and I want you to ask these folks if they are okay with knowing so many people who have suffered from those health conditions. (You can watch a video of this exact scenario being presented in front of a group of people at InspiredToBeHealthy.com)

This has become the new norm in America. Suffering from these conditions has become socially acceptable and even expected. I'm here to tell you that there is nothing normal about these statistics. Only in America is getting labeled and spending most of your life taking pills, and ultimately suffering from health conditions, normal.

Now I'd like for you to take this exercise one step further: **"If you were one of the many to raise your hand, I want you to slow down and think about the person that you knew who suffered. How was that person the day before he or she experienced or found out he or she had this condition? Better yet, how were they a week before? A month before? Even a year before?!"**

In most of the cases, these people were fine! They looked okay, and they felt normal. Heart disease and cancer do not happen overnight. It takes years and years to develop these conditions, however, because we "feel" fine and we "look" fine, we ignore all the warning signs along the way because we don't know any better. Cancer and heart disease rates in America continue to climb. It's getting ridiculous. Genetics have been used as a scapegoat for years now, meaning anytime someone becomes sick and there was no obvious cause, they (the medical system) would label the illness as "genetic" and insist there is nothing they (the patient) can do about it. The latest and greatest studies have shown that these life-threatening diseases have very little to do with genetics. In fact, less than 5% of any disease, condition, or syndromes are genetic related. Rather, what has been found is that these diseases are associated with the patient's lifestyle and environment.

The fact is, most parents raise their children in a similar fashion to how they were raised because it's all they know. A good example to get the point across is obesity. Let's say that Great Grandpa struggled with obesity and lived a poor lifestyle: ate fatty foods, drank sugary drinks, and didn't make exercise a rhythm in his life. He raised his son (Grandpa) in a similar, toxic, non-thriving environment, watching a lot of television rather than being active, snacking throughout the day, etc., and Grandpa ended up suffering from obesity as well. Now Great Grandpa suffered from obesity, Grandpa is currently suffering from obesity, and Dad followed in their footsteps and is obese. Does that Dad's child have to grow up and suffer from obesity?

If you want to play the genetics game and take the easy way out, then the answer is "yes" – this child has a slim chance of escaping the genetics of obesity. The idea behind that is just silly. The reality is if this child is raised in an environment of nutritionally deficit food, bombarded with sugary drinks, and dismisses physical activity all together, then more than likely, he will follow in their footsteps. On the flip side, if the child wants to take responsibility and break the cycle of unhealthy eating habits and decides to make time in his life to exercise, then the simple answer is "no," there is no reason why that son must suffer from obesity like the past generations. If the son were adopted by a family across the world, raised in a completely different environment with a completely different lifestyle, he could potentially end up as fit and healthy as a mule.

Does this have anything to do with genetics? Absolutely not! Being fit has nothing to do with genetics and everything to do with lifestyle and environment. Obesity is simply an obvious and easy condition to apply this too, but the reality is you can replace obesity with any health condition or disease and have similar outcomes if you're willing to change your environment and live a lifestyle that is congruent with your health goals. Don't get sucked into the system, there is a better way.

Mentoring Moment

Game Changer: Revisit the five-question quiz in this chapter, and allow the impact of the information to sink in. The easy and common thing to do is to ignore and laugh off the uncomfortable feelings of the health crisis we are currently experiencing. The reality of this emotional giant is overwhelming, and this will be the first of many bites as we eat this giant monster one speck at a time.

Own It: To get the most out of this chapter, take the principles that you learned and teach them to someone else. If you can't teach these principles, then you don't know them. If you don't know them, you're simply not going to be able to apply them to your life.

Go ahead! Take the next opportunity you have in front of a group of people, and apply the Application Exercise that you learned in this chapter!

2
Stressed Out America: We Have Created A Health Crisis

"As a people, we have become obsessed with Health. There is something fundamentally, radically unhealthy about all this. We do not seem to be seeking more exuberance in living as much as staving off failure, putting off dying. We have lost all confidence in the human body."
Lewis Thomas, The Medusa and the Snail, 1979

There is no such thing as Healthcare in America, there is only "sick-care." Our reactive healthcare system searches for problems when we're healthy and only cares for us when we are sick or broken. By some means, we have justified referring to this reactive, sick-care approach as healthcare.

So why is this happening? To be blunt: MONEY. There is no money in healthcare, there is only money in sick-care. Americans allow the pharmaceutical industry to take responsibility for their own health, and they label the human body as "stupid." The pharmaceutical companies took advantage of our crazy busy lifestyles and offered up something that the majority of us couldn't refuse: a simple quick fix... just take a pill. Take this pill, and you will feel better. Take this pill, and your numbers will come back into normal range. Take this pill, and you will feel happy again. These companies did this for a simple reason: CONTROL.

Let's take a moment to think of a newborn. After birth, who teaches this baby how to breathe? Who teaches the baby how to hold its head up? Did someone have to teach the baby how to nurse on a nipple so that it could feed from mom's breast? The obvious answer is "no," of course not, and that is because the human body has innate intelligence, meaning the body is smart and knows what to do.

Right now as you read this book, your heart is beating and allowing blood to pump through your entire body, your lungs are allowing you to breathe in the oxygen that your body requires to function, your eyes are blinking, perhaps you just scratched your leg or head without even thinking about it, and whatever you last ate is being broken down, digested, and turned into the energy you require to function while filtering and storing up the waste products so that you can get rid of them later today through urination or defecation. Our bodies are smart, and they will function the way they were intended to as long as there is no interference.

Designed to Be Healthy

"The human body is an incredible machine, but most people only get out of that machine what their mind allows them to."
Rich Froning

The human body is brilliant, and we are designed to be healthy. So, why then do we get ill, and what really happens to our bodies when we experience sickness? Let's take the common cold for example. Perhaps you get a fever, runny nose, cough, and maybe even vomit and experience diarrhea. Obviously, none of these are fun symptoms to encounter, but if we step back and really look at what our bodies are doing, we can make sense of these processes and learn to appreciate our bodies. When there is a foreign invader, something in our bodies that simply is not supposed to be there such as a virus, bacteria, etc., our bodies turn up the temperature to kill this thing, and we experience a fever.

Think of a fever as the body sending out all its soldiers to fight the virus or bacteria. The body's soldiers are fighting this mini-war and are working so hard they are breaking a sweat! When they work hard, you heat up – fever! The inconvenience of the non-stop runny nose is one more tactic our bodies use to get those foreign invaders out. The same goes with a cough, sneeze, and certainly with the ever so troubling vomiting and diarrhea.

Think about food poisoning, if you ate food that your body recognizes as poisonous – would you prefer your body to simply ignore this and allow the poison to cause more damage as it is digested? No. So your body is smart and says OUT! – as FAST as possible! Now you may not like how this "feels" but I can promise you do not want that poisonous food to stay in your body.

So really, these symptoms all come down to perception. All these perceived-as-problematic symptoms are occurring for a good, logical reason. Yet, what are we taught and trained to do by the pharmaceutical industry the minute we start to experience any one of these symptoms?

That's right, we are taught to STOP them.

Oh, and don't worry, there is a pill for every symptom. So, we take these medications, drops, and magic syrups to ultimately stop these natural processes from happening, all so that we don't have to "suffer." God forbid we let these symptoms slow us down and interfere with our busy lifestyles. So, we hinder our very own innate intelligence, and we chase the symptoms away just like we're taught to do. This act of ignorance for how the body works allows for the foreign invaders to stay inside of us rather than getting them out. Over time, as we repeatedly cover up the symptoms and avoid addressing the actual problem, our immune system continues to progressively weaken, but because we "feel" good, we have no issues with swallowing the pills for short-term gratification. The problem is you can only sustain this pattern for so long, and the short-term gratification that we are after turns into long-term pain and sickness.

Drugs are clearly not a good, long-term solution. As you continue to allow your immune system to progressively weaken, over time this will lead to an autoimmune disease where your body begins attacking itself. Autoimmune diseases are precursors to cancer, and as we have already discovered, the cancer rates in America are skyrocketing.

Now, clearly most of us never plan on being on a prescription medication for a long period of time. However, the reality is when a doctor prescribes a medication there is no game plan for ever getting you off the medication. Think about this situation, the drug itself is not actually healing anything, the drug is simply masking a symptom. Unless you have a game plan to heal whatever is causing the symptoms, which most people don't, you can expect to have to take the medications for the rest of your life. And the scary thing is your body adapts to the medication. So as your body adapts, the drug becomes less effective and then the doctor has to increase the dosage. Well, this increase in dosage can only happen so many times until you reach the maximum dosage allowed for that particular medication, and low and behold, you will have to be put on a different drug. This process has become routine in our country and has led to a major problem.

So, as you can see, the prescription of drugs is a vicious cycle, and quite frankly, this cycle is designed this way so that you will never get out. This cat-and-mouse game all comes down to the fact that there is no money in healthcare, there is only money in sick-care. If your body is not functioning the way it was designed to, then you are in this cycle, at the mercy of our broken healthcare system.

To be clear, when I say there is no money in healthcare, I mean there is very little money to be made from people who are healthy. It costs a few hundred dollars a month at most for someone to stay fit with a gym membership. It costs a few hundred dollars extra per week for a family to eat organic, non-GMO foods from the local grocery store. It costs less than a few thousand dollars a year for someone to maintain full, optimal function through chiropractic care. These are just a few examples of services that insurance companies won't cover to keep people healthy.

Insurance companies will, however, cover the six-figure surgeries, diagnosis imaging such as MRI's, CT's, x-rays, labs, and useless "regular checkups," all of which do absolutely nothing to keep you healthy. In fact, they all seek to find something wrong with you because, AGAIN, there's only money where there is sickness and disease. Our medical system is so corrupt it should be illegal. Oh, did I fail to mention that your insurance will gladly cover medications? Of course insurance will cover medications, because once you're on one, you'll have to be on others to combat the symptoms caused by the side-effects, and then those companies have you for life.

Lastly, please understand that I used the common cold in the example above because it's something that everyone can relate to. I want to emphasize that the common cold in the example above can be replaced with any symptom or health condition, including the top three killers that you learned about in chapter one. Often, people believe because their condition has some Big Bad Scary Name associated with it, they don't have a choice but to simply take the medications and have the medical procedures done. Our medical system does an excellent job of using scare tactics and presenting false truths.

Respect Your Symptoms

Nobody wants to be labeled. Nobody wants to be different and have to put up with the pain or discomfort of symptoms. But are symptoms so bad?

Remember, our bodies are smart. Just like when a newborn cries when something is wrong or when they want something, symptoms are your body's way of communicating with you. The cry of a newborn, especially if the baby's cry is persistent and frequent, can be extremely overwhelming, frustrating, and even exhausting, but this cry is how babies communicate. Your body is no different; it will communicate with you in several ways, and typically, that annoying or even frustrating symptom is your body's way of telling you that there's something so much bigger going on. Please don't down play your symptoms and simply cover them up. Just like a crying baby, a fire alarm, and all the other warning signs in your life, listen and respond appropriately. Taking action rather than relying on medication could save your life!

For instance, let's say you're driving your car and your check engine light turns on; you can only ignore the light for so long until finally, you decide you must do something about the warning. So, do you take your car to your local mechanic to see what's wrong and get it fixed, or do you just slap a piece of duct tape over the light so you can't see it anymore? You may be laughing at this, but the truth is that's exactly what we do with our bodies. Anytime we have a symptom - the check engine light turns on – and we simply mask the warning signs with drugs, medications, lotions, and potions. We don't fix anything. There is a pill for everything that gives a temporary fix so that we can get on with our busy lives and ignore what's truly going on. That's America's Healthcare system, and that's why as a nation, we continue to get sicker and sicker.

In fact, what do we call that cabinet in our bathrooms? You know, the mirrored cabinet that the doors swing open. Yes, a medicine cabinet. That's our mindset here in America. We have been taught and trained to think that having a medicine cabinet in our homes is perfectly normal. Now, am I healthier if this thing is chock full of prescriptions and medications or if it's empty? As a nation, we continue to go down this medicated road, (believing that these drugs keep us healthy) even though we know the side effects are downright scary and long-term effects do more harm than good.

Short-term Gratification vs Long-term Pain

"Have you more faith in a spoonful of medicine than in the power that animates the living world?"

BJ Palmer

Have you ever seen anyone walking around with a bag of medications, smiling and living the life of his dreams? Of course not!

Everyone knows that medications are not a good long-term strategy, yet doctors prescribe new medications to millions of Americans with absolutely zero intentions of ever getting them off those medications.

When you or your child is prescribed medications, this is the start of a vicious cycle that will lead to more drugs, injections, and eventually surgery. This cycle is absolutely crazy. I know we laugh about the drug commercials we see on television with all the outrageous side-effects because we know the situation is silly and almost unbelievable. Yet, we continue to take these pills where the side effects are worse than the condition they treat in the first place. The pharmaceutical companies have mastered the advertising component, getting us to believe that there is hope and selling us the dream. Listening to this false hope and empty promises is foolish. Now, I don't know about you, but for me, continuing down this path is madness.

Application Exercise #2

Are you aware that the United States is only one of two countries that allow for drug advertisements on television? I challenge you: the next time you're watching TV and you come across a commercial advertising a drug, do yourself a favor and close your eyes and simply listen. Closing your eyes will take away all the distractions, the smiling faces, grandpa shooting hoops with his grandson, mommy dancing with her precious daughter, people smiling and laughing in the background, and of course, the beautiful scenic views! Eliminate these visual distractions, and you will quickly notice that the first five to ten seconds of the commercial will introduce a drug that MAY help certain symptoms followed by another sixty to seventy-five seconds of all the possible side effects of the drug.

Why do we do this to ourselves?! The majority of the side effects rattled off are ten times worse than the symptoms the drugs are meant for in the first place!

There is literally a magic pill for every symptom, and rather than trying to figure out what's actually causing a problem, we take the easier, more convenient approach of trying to mask a symptom and cover it up with a drug. And the scary part is we all know that we shouldn't let ourselves get caught in this cycle, yet we continue to wait until our health has failed us, and we're left to make a healthcare decision out of fear, anger, or desperation. Have you ever said something out of fear or anger that you didn't really mean? Fortunately, an apology can get us out of that one, but your body may not accept an apology about your lost health. Every decision you make about your health sticks with you for the rest of your life, and rarely does anything good come from making a decision out of fear or anger.

The United States is experiencing an unsustainable disease burden – 130 million people today suffer from chronic illnesses. The vast majority of our two-trillion, healthcare dollars are spent treating chronic disease with drugs, injections, surgery, and experimental procedures. The current model is failing; we have more diagnosis, diseases, and syndromes than ever before. People have never been sicker. According to scholarly research, for the first time in the history of man, children born after the year 2000 are not expected to live as long as their parents. We are in a health crisis.

Health is being determined by pharmaceutical companies who send out sales reps to "educate" our doctors with the mentality that there is a pill for every symptom. Literally, these sales reps are being sent out with their verbal scripts, promotional materials, and a list of all the local doctors who they then treat to lunch in return for time to "educate" these doctors on the latest and greatest pills on the market. With all the new prescription drugs that are constantly introduced to the market, there's simply no way that doctors can keep up with the latest research.

And even if they could, "less than 15% of the medications that are prescribed here in the U.S. are backed by valid scientific evidence" (World Health Organization). The reality is we can make any study sound as pleasant or harmful as we would like. For instance, one study suggests that 22% of patients benefited from drug XYZ. Wow, that sounds wonderful huh?! Until you ask: what happened to the other 78% of the patients? Did they die?! If we plan to continue to base our health off of skewed studies, then we will continue to face this never-ending health crisis that we are in.

Even the commercials that we talked about earlier literally tell YOU to ask your doctor if drug XYZ is right for you. Doctors have gone from overseeing their patients' health to being the middle men and women. With properly prescribed medications being the number one killer in the United States, are drugs really the answer you've been looking for? Billions of dollars in profits are being made on these pills which are created in labs and sold to your doctor to pass along to you! Our healthcare system is complex; pharmaceutical companies want you to be overwhelmed and confused because then you have to keep running back to them for answers.

The doctors' job is to diagnose you because for every diagnosis, there is a medication. Think about that, the doctors' job is to find something wrong with you. And if there is nothing "wrong" with you, there is literally nothing they can do for you. The system will allow them to bend the rules a little bit, and if you're getting close to having something wrong with you (your numbers are getting close to being out of range), then they'll "proactively" put you on a medication.

The system is such a cookie-cutter approach treating every, single person the same. There is nothing personal or unique to the individual being cared for. Doctors today take all responsibility away from the patient so that the patient must rely on the system. For example, if a woman's blood pressure is 150 over 94, most doctors opt to give her a drug rather than explain to her why her blood pressure may be rising or encourage her to make a few lifestyle changes.

Perhaps she has high blood pressure because she is about 30 pounds overweight and doesn't work out and eats fast food every meal. The majority of doctors are not afforded the time to explain to the patient that if she were to lose a little weight, her joints would hurt less, and she would have more energy. And there's no time to explain that if she were to get her heart rate up three to five times per week, her heart would be strong enough to pump the blood through her body and her blood pressure would be normal. Instead, most doctors make it seem like she has bad luck and bad genes, and she's just going to have to learn to live with this condition and take the pills for the rest of her life.

Today that stops. If our doctors are unable to step up and help us live the long, healthy life that we deserve, then we'll just have to take matters into our own hands. After all, health is our greatest asset, do we really want to leave it in the hands of a broken system?

"The doctor of the future will give no medicine but will interest his patients in the care of the human frame, in a proper diet, and in the cause and prevention of disease."
Thomas Edison

Mentoring Moment

Game Changer: Revisit the "common cold" analogy in the "Designed to be Healthy" section of this chapter, and take some time to truly understand how the human body is brilliant! If you can comprehend that the power that made the body heals the body, you will learn to appreciate the benefits of the symptoms that you experience and learn to use them to your advantage for long-term health.

Own It: To get the most out of this chapter, take the principles that you learned and teach them to someone else. If you can't teach them, you don't know them. If you don't know them, you're simply not going to be able to apply them to your life. Please don't allow yourself to get sucked into the health crisis only to find yourself having to take medications to keep you sick for the rest of your life.

Go ahead! The next time you find yourself watching television, apply the Application Exercise in this chapter; keep an ear out for the drug commercials and listen to how insane the side effects are!

3

The Flexner Report: The WHY Behind Our Broken System

"Sometimes, I get the feeling that the pharmaceutical companies are sponsoring your symptoms."

Dr. Cotey Jordan

The first two chapters may have felt like a punch in the gut as we begin to unravel the reality of the crisis in our country. For those of you who are having a tough time digesting the information, this chapter will give you some of the details that will help you better understand why our healthcare system became what it is.

Medicine has become what it is today in large part due to one individual by the name of Abraham Flexner. In 1910, Abraham Flexner published the book, *Medical Education in the United States and Canada*, which is now known as the "Flexner Report." Abraham Flexner was not a doctor, but this school teacher and educational theorist from Louisville, Kentucky had a greater impact on modern medicine than anyone else.

Although institutions like Johns Hopkins already had contemporary principles in their work, most medical schools had not yet adopted these modern beliefs. If Flexner had not submitted his report that examined medical schools in the United States and Canada, healthcare as we know it would have most likely been fundamentally different.

For example, Flexner tried to clean up and standardize medical education with a system that focused on laboratory research, studies, and the patenting of medicine which would further supplement the entrepreneurs who financed and benefited from the 1910 *Flexner Report*: John Rockefeller, Andrew Carnegie, JP Morgan, among others.

Why were Rockefeller and others so interested in medical education? There are several theories, but one likely reason might have been these business men's interest in selling pharmaceuticals that began as by-products of petroleum refining. Whatever the reason, one thing is for sure, the combination of these mighty influencers gave federal legislatures the authority to create bureaucratic regulations and licenses that would stifle any and all medical facilities that did not comply with this regulatory superpower. In fact, according to the *Journal of American Physicians and Surgeons*, in less than fifteen years after the *Flexner Report* was published, the number of medical schools in the U.S. was cut in half, from 160 down to 80.

The *Flexner Report* paved the way for a medical monopoly that has only gotten worse as time goes on and continues to progressively worsen. Our modern system of healthcare has become a systemic force. There's a drug for every symptom, the drugs are patented, and the drugs are expensive and controlled by a small group of companies and government agencies. They have even portrayed the use of natural medicines as quackery!

I believe that the adoration of modern medicine and the addition of Western culture have placed our health in the hands of a greedy system that cannot make a profit when people are healthy.

Although this system has done many good things, the system is also largely blind to its sins and shortcomings. There are many good doctors and other medical professionals who try to do the best for their patients, but for the most part, modern medicine is deaf to the oath it wants to defend: the oath of Hippocrates. I believe that Flexner has paved the way for this reversal of whole-body health by making scientific research and specialized training the only desirable and credible approach to healthcare.

The *Flexner Report* brought to light a new and untapped way of making money from medical science without the expertise of health professionals outside the herd. Health experts, who were prone to natural healing, posed the greatest threat to this standardization, as they continued to demonstrate that nature provides what is needed to treat or prevent almost any disease. After all, you cannot patent a plant or an essential oil, but you can patent a molecule made in a laboratory that is very similar to the molecule in plants. If profit is what you want, and everything seems harmless, then you make money while doing "good" to people.

But there is a problem with this system. Drugs in general are not a good long-term strategy. The pharmaceutical success is not based on the effectiveness of the drug. This system is based on the number of profits these drugs can generate. Drugs do a good job of making us feel good but are only made to treat the symptoms and rarely treat the true cause of any disease. In addition, medications cause other, secondary symptoms and sometimes require additional medication to compensate for their harmful side-effects.

We live in a fast-paced culture where we NEED instant gratification. This system is absolutely perfect for the quick-fix model that most Americans seek yet is detrimental to the health of our country. We are headed into a massive health crisis.

Mentoring Moment

Game Changer: This chapter does a fantastic job of providing a brief introduction to the work that historically had the most impact on our medical system. Abraham Flexner's report, (along with the backing of the ultra-wealthy: John Rockefeller, Andrew Carnegie, JP Morgan) ultimately lead to the medical monopoly of today's modern healthcare system. Believing that our country has always had the best interest of the people at the forefront would be nice, but like many things in our great country's past, the health and wellness of our great nation has been compromised by the almighty dollar.

Own It: If you're one for details, dig deeper and do your own research on the school teacher from Louisville, Kentucky who was able to influence the entire medical education system. Back in 1910, the book Medical Education in the United States and Canada was published, and there have been updated editions published since.

4

Becoming Super Healthy is Not a Fantasy

"Don't wish it were easier wish you were better. Don't wish
for less problems wish for more skills. Don't wish for less
challenge wish for more wisdom."
Jim Rohn

People are designed to be healthy. We were designed to
function optimally so that we reach our fullest potential,
but something called "life" happens. Life comes along, beats us
up, programs us with limiting beliefs, and conditions us to avoid
any possibility of failure. In chapter one, you were introduced
to the reality of our broken healthcare system which served as
your wake-up call. The alarming statistics should not have been
much of a surprise to you as we are all surrounded by people
who are suffering from health conditions.

Chapter two demonstrated how our bodies are brilliant and
served to inform you how the symptoms we endure on a regular basis serve a beneficial purpose. If we can learn to respect
our symptoms and not merely mask them, we can avoid falling
into the treacherous trap of desiring short-term gratification
only to end up with long-term pain, sickness, and disease.

Lastly, chapter three served to provide an explanation of the WHY behind our broken healthcare system. At this point, you may feel as if you got hit with a fire hose of information that goes against everything that you thought you knew about our healthcare system. This feeling of resistance you are experiencing is natural. What you do with this essential information moving forward is what truly matters. We need people like you to stand up and share these principles so that we don't continue down this path of sickness and disease.

Now, I understand that looking at a global problem like this can be quite overwhelming. In fact, most people want to avoid the burden all together and completely ignore the situation because of its enormity. After all, you may feel helpless and wonder what impact you could possibly have on such a vast crisis. But let me ask you this: are you as healthy as you would like to be, and are your spouse, children, and friends as healthy as you'd like them to be? Maybe there is someone in your life right now that is really struggling. He or she is having a hard time getting well or staying well. Maybe he has tried everything, but nothing seems to help. Maybe it's a friend, a co-worker, or a family member that is experiencing this hardship. Or maybe it's YOU that's having this experience.

Well, I'm going to let you in on a little secret: you were designed to be healthy. We are all born with an Innate Intelligence that allows our bodies to function the way that they were designed to function. How to become super healthy is not something that is taught in our schools or colleges. In fact, because health conditions are so common these days and so emotional to talk about, we as Americans have made it socially acceptable to be sick and even suffer from diseases. Some people even protest against those who attempt to live a healthy lifestyle as if they're challenging the status quo and mocking the sick. We are all born with the gift of innate intelligence which is why our bodies are able to heal.

Basic biology, physics, and anatomy allow us to understand how the human body works from an inside-out reference point. The inside-out reference point proves the body's capabilities of functioning as long as there is no interferences from the outside to interrupt the body's natural processes.

Our healthcare has an outside-in reference point, and this backwards approach is why the system is broken. Rather than understanding how the body works and accepting its potential, our broken system takes the approach of advocating medications, injections, and surgery. All of these methods work from the outside world and affect the inside of the body. To think that man has outsmarted the natural inborn intelligence created by a Universal Intelligence is quite foolish.

I find it odd that our schools teach us how to read and write, how to do math and science experiments, how to memorize history and geography, and how to pass a test, but our education system never addressed or taught the subject of how to live a lifestyle that will keep us healthy and happy. Health and fitness seem to be a topic reserved for fantasies, movies, and super heroes. The majority believe that being super healthy is for the lucky ones, the rich, the people who win the genetic lottery, and the famously good-looking stars we see on television.

The reality is there are people who are becoming super healthy from all walks of life. In fact, most people who have made a major shift in their lives and began reaching their health goals are the ones who were told there was nothing left they could do. These people were sent home with no real solution, told they were to learn to live with their condition, and told they would have to rely on their medications for the rest of their lives. At some point (and we all get there), we decide that enough is enough, and we simply don't want to live like this anymore. I urge you and give you a friendly reminder that you don't have to hit rock bottom before you make your health a priority. In fact, I highly recommend you don't wait that long.

Application Exercise #3

In my office, we use a 3-Minute Health Questionnaire to get patients to see where they are and where they want to go. Take a moment now and answer the following questions as honestly as possible. Then, ask five of the closest people in your life to do the same. (You can download the "3-Minute Health Questionnaire" at InspiredToBeHealthy.com)

1. Do you want to be healthy? Yes / No / I Don't Care

2. What does it mean to be healthy? _____

_____

_____

3. Are you as healthy as you would like to be? Yes / No

If "No": What do you feel is holding you back? _____

_____

_____

4. In 20-30 years from now, would you like to be as healthy as your parents currently are? Yes / No / Maybe

If "Yes": Have you considered using them as mentors to help you live healthier? Yes / No

If "No": Do you feel that 20-30 years ago when your parents were your age, they wished to be in the current state of health they are in now? Yes / No

What are you currently doing to ensure that you don't end up like they did? _____

_____

_____

If you have kids, what are you currently doing for them to ensure they don't end up like your parents? _____

_____

_____

5. Do you personally know someone in your life who is/has suffered from either a heart attack, stroke, cancer, or diabetes? Yes / No   (Please circle which condition)

6. Based on your current knowledge of healthcare, which two or three of the following do you feel has the biggest impact on your health?

Germs   Medications   Environment

Lifestyle   Luck   Mindset   Genetics

What is Your Greatest Asset?

What is your greatest asset; what is the most important thing in your life? I should preface this question with there is no right or wrong answer. In fact, my father would quickly answer this question by proudly announcing that his 1972 Lemans is his greatest asset. He loves that car more than life itself!

So, take a few minutes to really think about this, "What is YOUR greatest asset?"

I recall when my wife, Amanda, was pregnant with what was to be our second child, and everyone wanted to know what gender our baby would be. My family, friends, patients, and military buddies would routinely ask if we were having a girl or a boy?

Amanda and I were the weird ones who chose not to find out what we were having! The further along in the pregnancy she got and the more her baby bump showed, the more people probed and commented. "Okay so you already have a daughter, I bet you're hoping for a girl!" "I would imagine you're looking to even things out with a boy and be done all together!" "You do know if you have another girl, you're going to have to have a third and shoot for that boy!"

As I recall, no matter how many times we were asked, my answer never changed. I always had the same response. I would reply, "We're just excited to be having another child! Truthfully, it really doesn't matter what the baby is as long as it's _____."

That's right, HEALTHY!

As parents, the only thing we're really ever after is for our children to be healthy and safe. All that mattered at that moment was that we were overjoyed to have a healthy addition to our family. At that moment, I whole-heartedly realized that health is my greatest asset: my own personal health, the health of my wife and kids, and the health of the people in my community. My wife and I truly didn't care what gender our baby would be. In fact, we didn't even realize we had a second daughter until over two minutes after baby Alex was born!

Isn't the health of you and your children your greatest asset? You could lose your job, house, cars, and all the money in the world, but if you lose your health, you have nothing. Many people get fooled by magazine covers and movies that imply success, wealth, and fancy materialistic objects are the most important things in life. Far too often, it takes a near-death incident or the death of a loved one before realizing that health is, in fact, our greatest asset.

If you never viewed health as your greatest asset in the past, I'd ask that you reconsider. The reality is you cannot be the best you and live out your life's purpose to the best of your ability if you are not healthy. You cannot be the best spouse, parent, friend, professional, or citizen that you're capable of being if you are not as healthy as you are designed to be. Your health is your choice. Choose to be healthy!

Investing in Your Greatest Asset

"Your health is an investment not an expense.
Although it will become an expense if you
don't take time to invest in it."
Ultra Healthy Mindset

Investing in health has been proven to be the greatest investment one can make. The top two stressors in America are health conditions and financial insecurity. Very few people recognize that these two issues are related. The number one cause of bankruptcy in America is medical bills stemming from health conditions that have taken years to develop. Health and finances are two delicate subjects that very few people feel comfortable speaking openly about. Addressing this issue head on and facing the reality of the emotional link in the middle of these two all-important topics is very important.

It is vital that you comprehend that there is no such thing as "health debt." Debt from being healthy simply does not exist. There is however, "sick debt," which can lead to financial disaster. Benjamin Franklin once affirmed, "An ounce of prevention is worth a pound of cure." Investing in your health now can save you hundreds and thousands of dollars over your lifetime and more importantly, allow you to avoid the top three killers in America: medications, cancer, and heart disease. Investing in your health throughout your lifetime will afford you the quality of life that many only dream about.

There are two mentalities you must be careful of adopting. First, avoid the mentality of becoming "debt free." Being debt free seems like the responsible thing to do, right? However, did you know that after years of digging deep and researching the habits and the mindset of people striving to achieve debt-free status, it was discovered that the important things in life were being neglected. Marriages suffered, family vacations were postponed or put on hold, kids participated in less sports and activities, etc. The examples are endless. Stingy spending habits on top of poor money management is negatively impacting the quality of life of the mass majority of Americans. We simply don't see that our becoming "debt free" mentality has affected our number one asset: our mental and physical health as well as the health of our kids.

If you're the type of person who is getting bogged down from the "debt free" mentality, the time is now to change your mindset. Giving yourself reasons of why you don't have the money to invest in yourself has to stop. Health is not something you budget for, it's something you invest in. If you honestly believed that your health was a top priority, then you would find the money to invest in yourself.

The second mentality you must be careful of adopting is on the opposite side the spectrum. This mentality is the "keeping up with the Joneses" mentality. Most Americans are walking around with their fancy, expensive smart phones, have satellite or cable television services, drive newer cars, and always seem to manage to come up with the money to eat out at a restaurant. If we live with the "keeping up with the Joneses" mentality, we are going to continue to feel the need to spend our money on things that really bring no joy or fulfillment to our lives. Again, we need to make our health a priority. What are your priorities? Are you trying to keep up with everyone else or are you making health a top priority? The truth is in your actions. Show me your checkbook and credit card statements, and I'll show you your priorities.

We're all guilty of having one or both mentalities! After all, isn't whipping through the drive-thru window and picking up a bag of one-dollar burgers and greasy fries more convenient than taking the time to get to the local market and spending the money for good, lean, healthy, organic beef and still having to go home and cook?! Isn't it easier to just act like nothing's bothering you as if any symptom will just go away on its own since your insurance provider won't cover the service or healthier options you need? Or better yet, take some magic pill or lotion to cover up your symptoms rather than addressing the underlying issue, all because your insurance provider truly knows nothing about you, your condition, or what type of care you need. But the company will gladly cover the cost of the one-size-fits-all drugs!

My hope is to bring these mentalities to your attention, so you can stop putting yourself second and make your health a top priority in your life. All it takes is one health crisis and all that hard work of becoming debt free is worth nothing. All the toys and gadgets you've collected are meaningless. The only thing that actually matters is your health. Churches around the country have acknowledged rapidly growing prayer requests with the top concerns addressing health issues. Start allowing your body to function the way God intended, and begin making your number one asset a top priority in life.

If you found out you had some rare disease and needed to come up with a large amount of money that you simply don't have for a lifesaving procedure, you would find a way to get the money. You would take out a second mortgage, perhaps sell your home, car, jewelry, or give up the much-needed phone, tv service, internet, etc. One way or another you would find a way! I suggest you find a way to invest in yourself now; investing now would be much easier and less expensive if you simply made your health a priority while you're alive, healthy, and having fun rather than waiting until a health crisis strikes.

If you're currently not as healthy as you would like to be, do something about your health now rather than waiting to hit rock bottom. It feels lonely down there, and you will feel hopeless. You'll find yourself asking, "What happened to me? How did I end up like this? Why did this have to happen to me?" You don't want to be in that place.

The time has come. Quit with the excuses. It's time to take action. The information in the upcoming chapters will transform your life and will empower you to take control of your health and the health of your loved ones.

Mentoring Moment

Game Changer: Health is not something you TRY to make room for in your budget; an investment in your health that MUST be made. Your health is your greatest asset. The number one cause of bankruptcy in America is medical bills. Don't make the same mistake that the bulk of Americans are making. You have two options; you can either invest in your health now, while you're young, busy, and having fun, or you WILL pay for health later when you become sick. If you choose the latter of the two, don't count on the quality of life that you dream about to be there for you during your retirement years.

Own It: To get the most out of this chapter, take the principles that you learned and teach them to someone else. If you can't teach them, you don't know them. If you don't know them, you're simply not going to be able to apply them to your life. Don't allow yourself to get sucked into the "debt free" mentality to the point of neglecting your greatest asset. Invest in your health today and for the years to come to ensure that you too can live to be super healthy.

Go ahead! Complete the Application Exercise in this chapter, and make note of the thoughts and feelings you encounter. Were you able to answer the questions effortlessly and with confidence? Were any emotions triggered thinking about your current state of health and what the state of your health could be if you follow in your parents' footsteps?

5

The Top 3 Reasons You're Not as Healthy as You Wish to Be

"Health is not a goal it's a lifestyle."
Ultra Healthy Mindset

After observing diverse lifestyles in eleven various countries, I began to see patterns of similarities and outcomes. The most common and obvious pattern that I became aware of is that there are three reasons why most people are not as healthy as they would like to be:

1. They have the wrong definition of health.

2. They lack personal responsibility.

3. They procrastinate and don't act.

Let's explore each reason in more detail, so you don't fall victim to these traps.

1. Wrong Definition of Health

"Health is a Journey, not a Destination."
Ultra Healthy Mindset

The majority of people that I ask would agree that they want to be healthy and stay healthy for the rest of their lives. Rarely do we see people walking around, hanging their heads in disappointment saying, "Man, I wish I were a little less healthy today!" Of course not! We all want to be healthy. So, if we all want to be healthy, yourself included, are you able to tell me what it is that you're currently doing for your health? Better yet, what is health?

If you're like most people, you're spinning right now, tripping on your words, and unable to answer the question confidently. The truth is if I were to go out into a public store or restaurant and pick ten random people to answer the question, "What is health?" I would most likely get ten different answers. Typical answers that I get include, "I'm healthy if I look good. I'm healthy if I feel good. I'm healthy if I work out, eat right, do yoga, count calories or steps, if I'm skinny, take vitamins, not sick, or simply when I'm happy or can get through the day without any issues."

To be clear, none of these are horrific answers. However, even though my question is very straightforward, very few people can answer it. And the people that do attempt an answer put their own little twist on the answer to match their idea of what they believe health to be.

The issue at hand is you simply can't be something you don't fully understand. The reason most people never achieve their health goals or become super healthy is because they simply don't have the information to be able to achieve health – they don't know what health even is. Since you can't be something you don't fully understand, let's start by defining what it even means to be healthy.

The definition of health is "the optimal function of your body; physically, mentally, emotionally, spiritually, and chemically." The keyword there is FUNCTION. Therefore, if you want to be healthy, your body needs to function to the best of its ability so that it can work the way it was designed to.

Being Fit vs. Being Healthy

"Being healthy and fit isn't a fad or
a trend. Instead, it's a lifestyle."
Ultra Healthy Mindset

If you would like to be healthy, age more gracefully, and avoid being a statistic of heart disease, cancer, or diabetes, you must be proactive with your health. We have all been taught and trained to base our health on how we look and how we feel.

The problem with this approach is if you're going to base your health on how you look and how you feel, you're only going to think about your health when you look bad or when you feel bad. And if you reach the point where you look and feel bad, there's a good chance it's too late to fully regain your health.

There is a huge difference between being fit - looking good and feeling good - and being healthy. There are people out there who are extremely fit, work out daily, and eat good clean organic, non-GMO foods. These folks are skinny, look great, and are shredded with muscle. They fuel their bodies with nutritionally dense foods while avoiding fast foods, junk foods, processed foods while minimizing sugar, wheat, and dairy in their diets.

There are hundreds of thousands of people like this living in the United States, and these are the people we put up on a pedestal and look up to as the ideal image of health. Unfortunately, many of these same fit people are suffering from chronic diseases and symptoms that are minimizing their quality of life. So, although they look good on the outside, they're suffering on the inside just like the majority of Americans.

The reason health conditions are so common here in America is because we have allowed the definition of health to evolve into something more convenient, something that takes the responsibility out of the people's hands and makes health something that can be "fixed" easily.

Your health is your greatest asset. Once you lose your health, getting it back is often impossible, and you're left with nothing. Health is much more than simply looking good and feeling good. If you truly want to be healthy, you must start with knowing what it means to be healthy.

HEALTH:
Your body functioning optimally the way it
was designed to - with zero interference.

2. Lack of Personal Responsibility

"Your health right now is a reflection of your past choices."
Ultra Healthy Mindset

The second reason people are not as healthy as they would like to be is because the responsibility of our own health has been taken away from us. We have been taught and trained that bad health is caused by bad luck, bad germs, and bad genes.

Therefore, there is nothing that we can do for our health except to hope that we are one of the lucky ones.

We've also been trained that we have to rely on someone else. For example, more and more Americans are suffering in the health care system because they are losing control over their health. If you're not in charge of your health, then someone else is. It's usually your insurance company or the pharmaceutical industry that's "in charge" of your health, and this situation is not okay.

Insurance companies tell your doctors how to treat you, and pharmaceutical companies tell your doctors what to give you. Somewhere along the way, our society taught us that doctors and nurses are supposed to keep us healthy rather than us taking responsibility for our own health and the health of our family.

From this point forward, you have no more excuses. You now know what millions of Americans don't; you know that health is your body functioning at an optimal level. You are now empowered to take your health into your own hands. Unless you step up and are willing to take on the responsibility of your personal health, you too will become a statistic.

I know with full certainty that anyone can become healthy, even super healthy, if he or she is willing to take action. Regardless of your current state of health, your family history, where you live, or what you do, you too can live a healthy lifestyle - I believe it's your responsibility to do so.

Your health is your responsibility and nobody else's: not your doctor's, not your health insurance provider's, and not even your spouse's. Your health is your responsibility.

Relinquish Your Health to No One

"The patient should be made to understand that he or she must take charge of his own life. Don't take your body to the doctor as if he were a repair shop."

Dr. Quentin Regestein

You give a large amount of your hard-earned money every month to have health insurance, and I understand you want to be able to use that insurance - you should be able to use it! Unfortunately, the number one cause of bankruptcy in America is medical bills and the majority of those people have "great" health insurance. Do health insurance companies really have our best interest when it comes to our health?

The reality is if you're relying on your Health Insurance to keep you healthy, you're in BIG trouble. Who at your health insurance company knows who you are and the daily stressors you endure? Who at your health insurance company knows the details of your health? Who knows about the intricacies of your condition or sickness? The obvious answer is "no one." The people at those companies don't know anything about you other than your policy number and a generic history, yet we are going to let them determine the type of care we are allowed. We often rely so heavily on our coverage that we convince ourselves to avoid the services and products that are truly in our best interest. If you allow your health insurance to determine your health, you will surrender all responsibility and your health will be determined by the very system that has lead us to the health crisis in America.

Your health insurance exists just as any other insurance you have. Do you really want to be able to use your life insurance tomorrow? Of course not, that would mean you're dead! Does your auto insurance pay for you to get an oil change? How about to get new tires or an upgrade to a stronger, faster engine? Of course not, so why do we expect this from our health insurance? The reality is we as Americans take better care of our cars and homes than we do ourselves. We will run our cars into the ground, and when they're all rusted out with 180,000+ miles, we'll trade them in for something new and better. Unfortunately, the situation is not that simple when it comes to our bodies. We beat our bodies up and run them into the ground, and by the time we realize what a poor job we have done taking care of them, it's usually too late and merely trading our bodies in for new ones is not an option. This is usually the point where we rely on our insurance to somehow magically restore our health. But health simply doesn't work that way.

Your health insurance is for health crisis. Crisis care involves emergencies such as major auto wrecks, traumas, serious burns, scary injuries, accidents, etc. The crisis care in America is world class and truthfully there's nowhere better to receive such care. However, when it comes to health, America struggles and puts little to no emphasis on long-term quality of life. Rather, Americans focus on the short-term gratification of temporarily relieving symptoms and feeling good as quickly as possible.

Most health insurances are not going to cover the services and products that are going to keep you healthy and allow you to function to the best of your ability: gym memberships, fitness coaches, supplements, maintenance chiropractic adjustments, health coaches, or even any type of nutritional education.

Are you able to walk into Whole Foods grocery store and flash your health insurance card to get a discount on organic food? Do insurance companies urge you to eat healthy and fuel your body with nutritious foods while avoiding processed, GMO, and addictive foods? Absolutely not! They do however cover drugs, surgeries, MRI's, CT scans, X-rays, etc. with their policies. The truth is your health insurance company does not have your best interests at heart. In fact, health insurance does not apply to healthcare; health insurance applies to sick-care - insurance only benefits you when something traumatic occurs or when you're sick.

If health insurance companies truly had your best interest in mind, they would go around to all the fast food joints and dis-enroll people who regularly eat at those places. They would mandate the use of gym memberships and strict food guidelines to those suffering from obesity. In fact, they would raise the premiums of those who do not work out regularly and those whose pantries are full of junk food. People who are not func-tioning to the best of their ability, eating appropriately, working out regularly, or investing in their greatest asset – their health – would be treated like smokers and alcoholics, and their premi-ums would be raised substantially. The mentality behind insur-ance companies would change drastically if health insurance were truly about the health of the people paying for it.

Ultimately, if you don't care enough to take responsibility for your own health, why should the insurance company care?

I want to reiterate this because it's that important and a huge problem here in America: Health insurance is meant to cover traumas and major medical issues. Health insurance is like life insurance, you shouldn't want to have to use it, but should feel at ease knowing it's there.

Unfortunately, nowadays the majority of people rely on their health insurance to keep them healthy, and if their health insur-ance doesn't cover a certain procedure or practice, these people don't even consider having that procedure to be a viable option, even if the procedure is the very thing they need. A major part of this issue is the cost of the premiums for health insurance... people pay big money for their insurance and they want to be able to use it.

How many times have you heard or spoken these words, "Do you accept my insurance?" "Will my insurance cover this?" "I can't go to Dr. XYZ because he's not an in-network provider." These statements showcase that your insurance company dictates the type of treatments you're able to seek, how long they will let you receive care, and who you can see to receive care.

For example, if you had two people (one had great insurance, one had no insurance), and they went to the emergency room, do you think they would get the same care? The sad truth is unfortunately not. Why? Because our healthcare system is no longer focused on what's best for the patient. Instead of being patient-focused, physicians are forced to care for you based on what insurance companies will and will not cover. No, this is not fair. But this situation happens every day.

To further emphasize my point, here is a quote from Medicare Guidelines, Section 2251.3: "Maintenance therapy include services that seek to prevent disease, promote health and prolong and enhance the quality of life, or maintain or prevent deterioration of a chronic condition. <u>Maintenance therapy is not medically reasonable or necessary and is not payable under the Medicare program</u>."

Does this sound like a healthcare system that has your best interest in mind? Don't let the lack of coverage by your insurance company keep you from being healthy! Also, don't allow your doctor's lack of time to educate you on a healthy lifestyle negatively impact your health. Take what they have to say and throw in your own common sense. Don't let scare tactics or false hope encourage you to put chemical stresses into your body. Address the problem head on, and if you're not getting the answers to your problems, keep searching until you do get logical answers that are going to address the weaknesses and vulnerabilities that are causing your health condition. Remember that your body is smart. Remove the interferences rather than just mask the symptoms, and give your body a fighting chance to take care of you.

Let me ask you a question: where do you see yourself in twenty, thirty, even forty years from now? Will you be the one heading towards the cruise ships or with the majority heading towards nursing homes? The choice is yours.

Your health is your responsibility. It's your greatest asset. Take complete responsibility for your health, and fight for your health no matter what. Your health is the most precious thing you will ever have in your life.

3. Procrastination

"Procrastination is the thief of health."
Ultra Healthy Mindset

The third reason most people are not as healthy as they would like to be is procrastination. We as Americans are experts when it comes to procrastinating. This talent has a lot to do with our lifestyles. The American lifestyle is go-go-go, now-now-now, how much can I get done, and please don't stress me out! This lifestyle and mindset contribute to the health crisis that we are currently in.

Because we live such a fast-paced lifestyle, we tend to downplay reality, convincing ourselves that our potential health conditions aren't a big deal. We put ourselves on the back burner, seeking a quick fix from popping pills to get us through the day so we can deal with the pain or symptom again tomorrow.

The problem is that symptoms are not really the problem - symptoms are a good thing. If we listen to our bodies when it communicates to us, we will have all the information's we need to be able to function at our peak level. Unfortunately, we chase symptoms instead of addressing underlying causes.

Let's face it, today we have access to more medications, procedures, vaccines, and injections than ever before, yet we are experiencing more sickness and have more diseases, syndromes, diagnoses, and health conditions than ever thought possible. The current system is failing.

You now have all the information you need to stop procrastinating. The upcoming chapters are going to introduce you to the Six Steps to Creating then Achieving Your 30-Year Health Goals & Living Super Healthy. These next chapters will guide you to stop procrastinating when it comes to your health. These Six Steps have taken people just like you to the next level and have given families the competitive edge in healthcare.

An obvious example would be a typical mother. If you're a mom (or the mom of the household) and your health fails you, is it worse for you or your family? When mom is worn down, frustrated, and out of commission, the entire family suffers.

That's just what moms do! They put everyone else's needs before their own. They learn to live with the daily overwhelm and exhaustion. The "off" feeling is their new norm. I must say what moms are capable of and what they do on a daily basis admirable, but this "norm" is not healthy.

Dragging our feet and thinking up reasons to put off our health conditions is both easy and common: not enough time, limited money, exhaustion, fear, my family comes first, unawareness, etc. These are called "reasons." Reasons make us feel good about not living up to our standards and help us justify our procrastination. In all reality, they are excuses. Excuses just sound too harsh and don't make us feel as good, so we stick with giving ourselves reasons. We know who we are, who we are becoming, and what we should be doing, so anytime we deviate from our core values, we are going to experience guilt, fear, and an entire assortment of emotions.

Additionally, many of us have an extremely limited mindset about health, and we believe the excuses we tell ourselves. While I do understand that we are all "busy" and that money does not grow on trees, I also know that every single person in this world is limited to the same twenty-four hours a day, and many are able to find the time and the resources to make their health a top priority. Regardless what you think is holding you back from being healthy, let's get rid of the reasons and the excuses, and let's start making yourself a priority.

Many people do not have health as one of their top priorities until they have lost their health, and then regaining that health becomes their number one priority. This circumstance is due to the reactive mindset that we adopt from our flawed healthcare system we are forced to participate in.

Don't let anyone tell you it's not possible. Family, acquaintances, leaders... don't let them tell you that what you're trying to do for you and your family is not possible. You don't want to be that person 20 years down the road who is bitter, miserable, or angry at the world, wishing you would have done something differently. There are endless studies out there that show that when people are laying on their deathbeds reflecting on their lives, regret is what's on their minds. They regret what they wish they had done.

This is essentially why the six-step system that you will read about in the upcoming chapters was created – so that you're able to live your life out to the fullest while experiencing an amazing quality of life and having fun doing so.

Mentoring Moment

Game Changer: Answer the following questions...

- What is Health?

- What is the difference between being HEALTHY and being FIT?

- What are you doing today that demonstrates you are taking personal responsibility for your health?

- What choices have you recently made that impacted your health negatively?

- Why did you make those choices?

- Regarding your last answer... are those Reasons or Excuses?

Own It: Reasons are no better than excuses. Reasons are generally softer and make you feel better for not doing what you said you were going to do. Buck up and take ownership; your reasons are your excuses! If you can take ownership of them, you can beat them.

To get the most out of this chapter, take the principles that you learned and teach them to someone else. Ask these same questions above to the people in your life and discuss the answers with those people. If you can't teach these principles, you don't know them. If you don't know them, you're simply not going to be able to apply them to your life. If you don't plan on applying this to your life, then really what are you even doing here?

Go ahead! The next time you find yourself providing reasons why you're procrastinating, call them what they are and address your excuses immediately. You don't need them! They're not who you are!

6
Stress Attacks the Weakest Part of the Body

"Illness is the result of imbalance. Imbalance is a result of forgetting who you are. Forgetting who you are creates thoughts and actions that lead to an unhealthy lifestyle and eventually to illness.... Illness can thus be understood as a lesson you have given yourself to help you remember who you are."

Barbara Brennan

We all live under this umbrella of life called "Stress." No matter your age or the stage of life you're currently at, stress will always affect you. The reality of stress is that it attacks the weakest part of the body. When we have a ton of stress in our lives (kids, work, money, relationships, lack of sleep, etc.), what happens is that stress builds up and leads to a number of different health conditions. Every health condition known to man is in some way caused by stress. And that's because stress attacks the weakest part of the body.

The urgent problem we face is that very few Americans have a clue of what the weakest parts of their bodies are. These weaknesses and vulnerabilities, compounded by the daily stresses of life, make our bodies progressively weaken and degenerate, leading to poor health conditions. In my professional opinion, everyone must be checked to know and fully understand where they have weaknesses and vulnerabilities in their bodies, so they can give these areas the attention needed to remove the interferences and allow their bodies to function to the best of their abilities.

If your intentions for reading this book are to be proactive because you are truly serious about living a healthy lifestyle and maintaining your health as you age, understanding how the human body works and how stress affects the body is essential.

You literally have two options to proactively manage your stress. First, you can learn to consciously manage your stress on a regular basis, and second, you can put the time and energy in to become in-tune with your body, learning where you're weak and vulnerable and ultimately strengthening these areas to ensure that you can better handle the stress.

My suggestion is that you do both. I will say however that the latter of the two is by far the more effective of the two. Unless you learn to manage your stress twenty-four hours a day and seven days per week, which I would argue to be next to impossible for anyone living the American lifestyle, your body will progressively weaken and degenerate, leading to you aging a lot less graceful than you would like.

In the upcoming chapters, I will teach you the keys to removing the interferences as well as managing your stress so that you are able to reach your peak state of health and live the super healthy lifestyle that you're capable of. But first, let me give you a glimpse into how a common monkey-wrench in your daily routine can not only impact your day but impact your health.

Let's say you start your day pouring yourself a cup of coffee. You then get started on your to-do list and... BOOM... the phone rings or the baby is crying or the kids are making a mess all over the floor. In other words, the chaos begins! And you begin reacting to situations. You're now working on someone else's agenda. Someone needs your help, and you give it to him. You're in a fix-it mode.

So, what happens in the body? First, your body immediately shifts the blood flow in the brain to the hindbrain, where your fight-or-flight mechanism is controlled. Then, your cortisol and other stress hormone levels increase, and you begin to get irritable and feel stressed out.

Stress is natural in the body, but it's not meant to be sustained. When you have a morning like this and deviate from your original game plan for the day, you crash in the middle of the day because the adrenaline running through your veins all morning finally dissipates and leaves you feeling tired and worn out.

This stress leads to other stresses. It's a snowball effect. And if you have other people, family, or co-workers who depend on you, I feel for you because far too often you have days like this. You are over-tasked and underappreciated (and let's face it, who doesn't want to be acknowledged for all that you do and appreciated for who you are?!) And when you don't get that attention you know you deserve, you get even more down on yourself and exhausted. It's a vicious cycle that no one should have to go through, but unfortunately, most do.

Stress Attacks the Weakest Part of the Body

There are four types of stress we all experience on a daily basis: physical stress, mental stress, emotional stress, and chemical stress. Let's look at each type of stress and some examples, so you can start pinpointing the stressors of life and begin to manage those stress triggers.

Physical Stress: Poor posture is a physical stress that plagues the majority of Americans. People who sit at desks all day every day are what I call "corporate athletes." Corporate athletes are hunched over for eight to ten hours a day, putting stress on their entire bodies, and they do this for a 30-40-year career. These folks often have poor posture because the hunched-over, seated position becomes their new normal, and the impact this posture has on their nervous systems rarely leads to these folks retiring with their bodies functioning optimally. Postural distortions are often the result of repeated physical stress.

Examples of Physical Stress: poor posture, auto accidents, sports trauma/injury, exercising with bad form, repetitive lifting or motion, yard work, sitting in a forward, flexed position for 20 minutes or longer.

Mental Stress: Let's face it, if you have a job, attend school, or are a stay-at-home-mom, you are mentally stressed. There's simply not enough time in the day to get everything on your to-do list done, and nowadays, you're expected to do more with less. This lifestyle is not only mentally exhausting, it's extremely stressful as well.

Examples of Mental Stress: work, school, time management, anxiety, depression, expectations.

Emotional Stress: If you've been married or in a relationship for any length of time, you've experienced emotional stress. You may have the perfect partner, but being able to meet each other's emotional needs 24/7 is next to impossible. Disagreements and even discussions often lead to the rise of cortisol levels, putting our bodies on high alert. And if you have kids, well then you already know there will be stress along the way. The number one emotional stress is money. There's simply never enough of it, and no one has been able to create the money tree for us all to plant in the back of our yards.

Examples of Emotional Stress: marriage/personal relationships, raising a family, work, financial obligations, driving in traffic, economic concerns.

Chemical Stress: Chemical stressors are the leading stressors we face here in America. Eating healthy here in the States is next to impossible, as we've been inundated with convenient foods such as GMO's, processed foods, fast foods, and of course the endless junk foods on the market. On top of that, the majority of Americans are putting chemical toxins into our bodies every single day via sugar, caffeine, medications, tobacco products, and alcohol. Breakfast usually consists of cereal (a sugar bomb) for kids and a coffee loaded with sugar and dairy for adults. If we eliminated the chemical stress here in America, that change alone would cut down our diseases and sickness by over 50%.

Examples of Chemical Stress: medications, fast food, processed foods, drinking tap water, breathing air pollutants, cleaning supplies, alcohol, tobacco, sugar, wheat, dairy.

The Law of Life

We live in a universe in which there are laws. A law simply states that if ABC happens, the outcome will be XYZ, no matter what. Regardless what you think or believe to be true, or even if you like it or not – these consequences are absolutely going to happen. If a law is broken or not followed, there will always be an outcome or a consequence.

Let's start with a law that we're all very much so familiar with: the Law of Gravity. Let's test out this theory. If I were to grab hold of a pen, extend my hand in front of me, and then let go of the pen, what do you think would happen?

What if I told you that I whole heartedly do not believe in gravity? Not only do I not believe in gravity, I think that the entire idea of gravity is stupid. Would this alter your answer and the outcome of what happens to the pen after I let go?

Of course not! Because the Law of Gravity exists, and regardless of my thoughts, feelings, or beliefs, the pen will clearly hit the ground after I let it go. The same goes for falling out of a tree. If someone slips, regardless if they're nice or mean, rich or poor, attractive or unattractive, the results will be the same, and that person will fall and hit the ground.

I'd like to introduce you to a little less known law called the "Law of Life." The Law of Life is a law of nature; it is as impartial and impersonal as the Law of Gravity is. It is precise, and it is exact. The Law of Life states that optimal health exists when the human body is functioning at 100% of its potential with zero interference. The law suggests that a person will experience health and ultimately a pleasant quality of life as long as his or her body is FUNCTIONING to the best of its ability.

So, let's test this theory as we did with gravity. What would happen if someone's head was cut off? That person would absolutely die. How about if the nerve root to his heart was cut? Again, that person would certainly die, not 70% of the time, but 100% of the time, therefore, making this a law!

Let's give a less extreme example. Let's say someone's body was only functioning at 60% of his capability due to interference. Would this person be experiencing optimal health? Absolutely not! In fact, if his body was only functioning at 60% of his max capability, then I think it would be safe to say that there would be a high probability for this person to experience negative health conditions – symptoms, syndromes, or disease. Wouldn't you agree?

This is a very powerful piece of information. In fact, that information is life changing! As you just learned, the definition of health is your body functioning optimally the way it was designed to – with zero interference. So, if health is optimal function, the next question we must be asking is, "What controls every single function of your body?"

The answer is the brain. In order for the brain to be able to control every single function of the body, the brain must be able to communicate with the entire body so that the body can function the way the body was designed to. So how does your brain do this? Your brain sends life energy through your spinal cord. Your spinal cord is your lifeline. It's like a river. Your spinal cord takes the energy from your brain, through your spine, and out hundreds of thousands of nerves to every single nook and cranny in your body. All of your vital organs, all of your major muscles, and every single gland, tissue, and cell in your body are totally dependent on this energy to keep you alive and healthy. As long as there is free flow of energy from your brain to the rest of your body via your nervous system, you are following the Law of Life, and therefore, experiencing optimal health. If there is any interference whatsoever with the flow of the energy, then the Law of Life is being broken, and as with any law, there are consequences.

These consequences typically come in the form of symptoms. As stated in chapter two, symptoms are not the problem, they're our body's way of communicating with us, expressing that something is wrong. Because we have been taught and trained to treat symptoms, we rarely address the actual cause and we continue living with our bodies in a state of pain or tiredness, breaking the Law of Life. As the interference of the energy worsens, our condition, and ultimately our health, progressively weakens and deteriorates.

Whether you believe in the Law of Life or not, like it or not, or even understand it or not, this is simply how the body works. The nervous system is the master system of the body; the nervous system controls every other system (immune system, digestive system, cardiac system, etc) in your body. If there is any stress or interference to your nervous system, it is physically impossible for your body to be functioning to the best of its ability.

Here is one more example of the Law of Life at work and how it affects you and your loved ones: someone you care about runs in the house screaming and yelling in pain, and he doesn't know what to do. He just fell off his bike, and he scraped his knees and elbow. There's blood everywhere! What would you do? Obviously, you'd jump up and help him! You'd calm him down, get something to wipe off the blood, and begin cleaning up the cuts. You'd then get some Band-Aids to keep the cuts clean and help stop the bleeding.

So, my question for you is this: a week from now when the cuts are fully healed and perhaps there are scars, was it the Band-Aids that healed the cuts?

The answer is "no." The body healed the cuts. This is a perfect example of the Law of Life. Except in rare occurrences when a person as hemophilia or another blood disorder that doesn't allow his or her body to clot normally, the body will take care of the cuts.

I'd recommend treating the Law of Life like the Law of Gravity; you can spend the next decade trying to figure the Law of Life out, mastering the concepts, or you can leave that up to the experts and just know that it's there and that it does exist. You will be healthy if you allow your body to function at 100% and not allow any interferences to bring you below 100%. Obviously, the lower that number goes, the less your body is functioning optimally and the more health conditions you will experience. This will eventually lead to disease.

Application Exercise #4

Now that you understand how stress attacks the weakest part of the body and leads to symptoms, complete the Personal Stress Assessment below to get a better idea of which forms of stress impact you the most and how they may be affecting your overall health. (You can download the "Personal Stress Assessment" and "Symptom Survey" at InspiredToBeHealthy.com)

Circle the forms of STRESS that you have experienced:

Physical Stress:

- Poor Posture

- Auto Accidents

- Sports Trauma / Injury

- Technology Usage

- Repetitive Lifting or Motion

- Yard Work / Manual Labor

- Poor Quality of Sleep

Mental Stress:

- Career

- School

- Time Limitations

- High Expectations

- Financial Instability

Emotional Stress:

- Marriage

- Kids

- Work

- Financial Obligations

- Driving in Traffic

- Economic Concerns

- Personal Relationships

- Lack of Emotional Support

Chemical Stress:

- Medications

- Fast food

- Processed Food

- Drinking Tap Water

- Breathing Pollutants – Air / Cleaning Supplies

- Alcohol or Tobacco Use

- Sugar / Wheat / Dairy Consumption

Circle any SYMPTOMS you've experienced in the last 6 months:

- Headaches
- Migraines
- Sinus Problems
- Allergies
- Mood Swings
- Depression
- Carpal Tunnel Syndrome
- Digestive Problems
- Asthma
- Restless Leg Syndrome
- Leg Pain
- Fatigue
- History of Cancer
- Female Disorders
- Chronic Colds

- Tension Between Shoulders
- Excessive Irritability
- Lower Back Pain
- Mid Back Pain
- Upper Back Pain
- Neck Pain
- Anxiety
- Chronic Diarrhea
- Dizziness
- Trouble Sleeping
- Loss of Appetite
- Chest Pressure
- Numbness / Tingling in the Arms / Hands / Feet
- Fibromyalgia

Stress attacks the weakest part of the body. If you are experiencing symptoms, you can rest assure that there are weaknesses and vulnerabilities in your body. Think about the stressors that you endure on a daily basis and how they can be contributing to the symptoms that you are experiencing. Remember that symptoms are not the problem, they are simply your body's way of communicating with you.

Your Spine Protects Your Life Line

Take a second to think about how amazing your body is. At this very minute, your brain is sending life energy through your spinal cord to all parts of your body. As you're reading this, your eyes are blinking, your lungs are allowing you to breath, your heart is pumping blood throughout your entire body, your stomach is digesting whatever you ate earlier, among a gazillion other things that your body is doing without you even thinking about it. Could you imagine if you had to think about all these processes while you're trying to read? Having to tell yourself to swallow, breath, blink, scratch, heartbeat, breath again, eyes keep moving so you can continue to read. Obviously, that would be impossible! With all the processes and responsibilities that your body has to take care of, this is the importance of understanding the Law of Life and ensuring that your body is functioning to the best of its ability.

To understand the importance of your spine, you must recognize that your spine has two functions. First, the spine supports and holds us up right. This is called your posture. You can tell a lot about somebody's health based on his or her posture. The second function of your spine is to protect your spinal cord. Similar to how your skull protects your brain, your spine protects your spinal cord. A healthy spinal cord is essential when it comes to your overall health.

Let me tell you why the spinal cord is so important. Because the brain controls every single function of the body and the brain does this by sending life energy through the spinal cord, it's essential that the twenty-four bones that make up your spine are properly aligned to protect your spinal cord. Your spine is like a river; it takes the energy from the brain, through the spine, out the nerves to every single cell in your body. All of your vital organs, major muscles, and glands are totally dependent on that energy to keep you alive and healthy.

Due to certain stresses in life, some are sudden and some over time, the individual bones that protect your spinal cord shift out of place. These shifts are called "vertebral subluxations." Subluxations block the energy from being able to pass through the spine and out the nerves. This interference causes your body to break down because your body is unable to function optimally.

Over time, this condition progressively worsens, and your body ends up in a state of dis-ease, which our medical system likes to call disease so that they can label us, diagnose us, and give us the new and improved drug to take. We are all very well informed that there is a drug for every symptom. Although there are a times and places for medications, drugs are not a good long-term strategy. And yet, the majority of Americans are prescribed medications with zero intention of ever getting off the drug.

In addition, subluxations will also weaken and distort your posture. Your posture is the window to your spine and nervous system. As already mentioned, you can tell a lot about someone's state of health based on his or her posture. Often time, people with poor posture will have a noticeable head tilt, uneven shoulders, appear rotated, or sit and walk around hunched over because they have a weak and distorted spine. These people are often in a lot of pain or experience symptoms and conditions from organ failure that our medical system can't explain. It's important to note that this situation very often occurs in kids who are young, vibrant, outgoing, and who look good and feel good. Because stress attacks the weakest part of the body, these are usually the kids who grow up to have major health conditions and diseases.

It is impossible for anybody to function to the best of his ability if he has a weakened posture caused by a subluxation in his spine because the subluxation causes constant stress on his spinal cord. Our flawed medical system pays little to no attention to the flow of life energy from the brain to the rest of the body, but instead chases symptoms and prescribes drugs for every problem in hopes to make you temporarily feel better rather than addressing the actual cause of the problem.

The wrong definition of health is by far the number one reason why people are not as healthy as they would like to be here in America. It's not even the people's fault. We have all been taught and trained to believe that health is this idea of looking good and feeling good, and that health is based on luck, genetics, and everything else that is out of our control. I would recommend reading this chapter over and over until you fully understand what "health" really means. Understand and embrace the Law of Life, the true definition of health (not America's definition of health), the difference between being fit and being healthy, and how stress in your life is affecting your overall health right now as well as the impact stress will have on your quality of life as you age.

Mentoring Moment

Game Changer: Stress attacks the weakest part of the body, causing uncomfortable symptoms and ultimately leading to sickness and disease. Stress is not going anywhere any time soon, so the time is now to learn to better manage your stress. Personally apply the Law of Life and watch your current state of health significantly change and ultimately lead to a better quality of life.

Own It: To get the most out of this chapter, take the principles that you learned and teach them to someone else. If you can teach and give examples of physical stress, mental stress, emotional stress, and chemical stress, then you will be able to own those examples. You will be more aware of them in your life and better suited to be able to handle your stress by applying the Law of Life. Invest in your health today and for the years to come to ensure that you too can live to be super healthy.

Go ahead! Complete Application Exercise #4: Personal Stress Assessment, and make note of which forms of stress impact you most and how they're impacting your overall health. Have the people closest to you in your life take the assessment as well, and discuss their answers with them.

PART 2

How to Create an
Extraordinary Life Using
the Knowledge, Tools,
and Rituals of the
ULTRA HEALTHY

7

The 6-Step Sequence to Extraordinary Health

"You know you are on the right track when
you have no interest in looking back."
Ultra Healthy Mindset

People need hope. People need to be inspired. People want something to admire, something to believe in, and some-one to look up to. Hope is an important piece of wholehearted living. I always thought of hope as a warm feeling of optimism and possibility. I was wrong.

Hope is not an emotion. It's a way of thinking. It's a cognitive process. Emotions play a supporting role, but hope is really a thought process. Hope happens when you can set realistic goals, figure out where you want to go, and then have the ability to achieve those goals.

The Six Steps that are laid out in the upcoming chapters of this book will walk you through this very process and are where you'll begin your personal journey beyond symptoms and help you develop your very own Roadmap to Extraordinary Health. Somewhere throughout this process, you will have a break-through and become empowered to take your health into your own hands. I have zero concerns when or where this breakthrough will happen, but I assure you it will happen.

Health consists of four components: Function, Food, Fitness, and Fun. I call these the "Core Four." If you truly want to be healthy, you need to have good habits and rhythms in all four of these areas. By simply lacking in even one of the Core Four, you will lose the ability to reach your maximum potential and the opportunity to experience extraordinary health.

As you begin your journey beyond symptoms, I will lead you through a six-step sequence that will guide you and keep you focused, moving you closer to extraordinary health and the person you are destined to be.

This six-step sequence is designed specifically so that anyone can navigate through the sequence at his or her own pace while taking leaps and bounds in his state of health. The Core Four will be addressed along this journey, and you will be encouraged to pick and choose strategies to develop your very own roadmap to get you living the lifestyle that will ultimately lead to extraordinary health.

The Six Steps are listed below and have a brief synopsis of what they entail. Go ahead and familiarize yourself with the Six Steps below before we dive in and begin your transformation.

Step 1: Mindset – Focus & Make the Decision

Step 2: Motivation – Creating and Achieving Your Health Goals

Step 3: Strategy - Design Your Ideal Lifestyle

Step 4: Accountability - Build a Healthy Environment

Step 5: Take Action – Develop Self-Discipline

Step 6: Celebrate & Refocus – Living Your Ideal Lifestyle

Step 1: Mindset – Focus & Make the Decision

You are where you are health-wise because of who you are and the decisions you have made in your life up until this point. If you are not satisfied or would simply like to improve yourself, then you have to take action. If you want something to change then you are going to have to change.

Mindset is all about how you think. If you change your thoughts, you change your actions. If you change your actions, you change your habits. If you change your habits, you change your life. And if you change your life, you can change the lives of the people around you.

One of man's greatest fears is failure – not being good enough. If you can recognize this fact, embrace it, and use this fact to benefit you, you'll quickly see that failure leads to greatness. We learn from our mistakes, and we tend to do things better. The problem is not when you fail, the problem is when you quit because you failed. The number one reason people fail is because they don't have a compelling reason to continue trying.

Learning how to control your mind and how to think at a higher level will have many additional benefits in your life. Having the right mindset will improve your relationships, your health, your financial future, your outlook on life, and much more.

Step 2: Motivation – Creating and Achieving Your Health Goals

The purpose of a goal is to motivate you. Goals simply get you to take that first uncomfortable step towards something that you want, but you're either scared or uncertain as to how to go about achieving what you want.

Goals are absolutely essential to bettering yourself in any area of life, and this idea is especially true when it comes to health and fitness. Yet, less than 85% of people actually take the time to set goals and write them out. They have no idea what they want in life. This fact plays a large role in the fact that over 70% of Americans are dissatisfied with their current health.

Most people believe that they are not as healthy as they can be simply because they lack the motivation. And that's simply not true. If you feel that others are successful because they're motivated and that you're just lazy, the reality is you're not lazy; you just have impotent goals. You have got to set goals that drive you and that have real power behind them.

Pain is often what gets us started and pleasure is typically what keeps us going. Your short-term goals will be pain-based to help you jump start your success, and your long-term goals will be pleasure-based to help you keep going when times get rough or you begin to lose focus.

You need to stay focused. You need to work on yourself every single day. This six-step process, along with the strategies provided for the Core Four, are what's going to keep you on target and accountable.

Step 3: Strategy - Design Your Ideal Lifestyle

With our Healthcare system exposed, the definition of health established, and your life purpose defined, take the time to build a roadmap to get you where you want to go. If you intend on experiencing extraordinary health and aging gracefully, you're going to need a strategy to do so.

Health and fitness are often overwhelming and complicated subject matter. The good news is that health doesn't have to be complicated. As mentioned previously, there are four components that determine ones state of health; I refer to these as the "Core Four." In order for you to be able to achieve your maximum state of health, you will be required to be strong in all four of these principles. Your personal health goals will determine which area receives the most emphasis when it comes to building your Roadmap to Extraordinary Health.

The Core Four are simply the breakdown of your lifestyle. There are several strategies that you will be able to pick and choose from to optimize your capabilities in each of the four areas. Here is a brief rundown of the Core Four.

1. Function: When your body is functioning optimally, it is working the way it was designed to – with zero interference. The brain controls every single function of the body. The brain does this by sending life energy down through your spinal cord and out hundreds and thousands of nerves to the vital organs, muscles, glands, tissue, and cells in your body. Incorporating a strategy or system that will strengthen, protect, and remove/avoid any interference to your brain, spinal cord, and the rest of your nervous system is absolutely vital.

2. Food: The purpose of eating is to fuel the body, to give our body the energy it needs to perform its daily functions. Your body is your temple. Don't fuel your body with garbage. Your temple deserves a solid foundation. Strong food leads to a strong body. A strong body leads to a strong mind. If you have a strong mind, you will be a strong human!

3. Fitness: Fitness plays a vital role in overall health. To be clear and to reiterate, there is a huge difference between being fit (looking good and feeling good) and being healthy. The purpose of fitness is to provide you with strength, mobility, flexibility, and cardiovascular potency. Ultimately, what you choose to work on doesn't matter, as long as you're doing something. All forms of exercise work as long as you're willing to put in the work. You have to enjoy whatever form of physical exercise you choose, otherwise there is very little chance that you will stick with an exercise routine and incorporate it into your lifestyle.

4. Fun: The purpose of life is to experience happiness. The opposite of happy is not unhappy or sad but boredom. If you find yourself regularly bored in life, you're clearly not as happy as you could be. Happiness is a choice. You can choose to be happy or you can choose to be miserable. The more you strengthen your mindset, the less limitations you will encounter and the more empowered you will be to live happily ever after. When it comes to your health, you need to have fun on a regular basis if you are to experience extraordinary health. After all, laughter and fun are the best medicine. We will incorporate some strategies that will give you permission to have fun and ultimately experience joy on a regular routine basis.

There's no one single principle that has the capability to make you as healthy as you would like to be. There is no quick fix or shortcuts to experiencing extraordinary health. Building your strategy is an essential step during your journey beyond symptoms.

Step 4: Accountability - Build a Healthy Environment

The top factors determining health are lifestyle and environment. Look beyond all the noise and confusion about health, and you will discover a select group of people who have created super healthy lifestyles.

Don't do what most people do and try to fit into your current environment. Do not limit yourself. You were born to be healthy. You were born to be excellent. You were born to make a difference. Surround yourself with people who see greatness in you.

If you're okay with being average, then you're going to end up like the average American and when it comes to health this is not a good thing. Choose to be better than average. Surround yourself with people who are on the same mission as you are. Cut off the people who are not on the same mission as you are. Yes, they will be upset. Yes, they will send you nasty emails and have nasty words for you. They may even make nasty comments on your social media feeds. However, I want you to know that this is a small sacrifice for the huge impact you will have on the world.

Growth happens naturally in the right atmosphere. If you know exactly what you want to be, you have to surround yourself with the people, places, and things that will help you get there. Surround yourself with people who are already like who you want to be. Surround yourself with the material objects that will support you and allow you to reach your goals. You have to surround yourself with positive people. There is too much negativity in the world we live in, and you will constantly be bombarded by this negativity if you don't plan ahead and create your own environment.

Step 5: Take Action – Develop Self-Discipline

Discipline does not have to be hard. Discipline does not have to be terrible. Discipline can be fun and joyful. Finding the joy in discipline goes all the way back to mindset. If you believe that discipline is a negative thing, you're probably never going to have it. People who have mastered discipline have shown that you can be disciplined and have fun while cultivating that skill.

The more disciplined you become, the more excellence you will experience in every aspect of life. Excellent people do things a little differently than the average Joe. They show up early, they move differently, they carry a confidence that commands respect. And whether you want the attention or not, people notice this difference, and they look at you, wondering what is it that you do differently. So, continue to train that discipline muscle, and you will notice changes in all area of your life. The only discipline that lasts is self-discipline.

Along with discipline, you will develop other important traits, values, and skills while working towards your health goals. You can use these same skills and values in other areas of your life. I promise that you will become more disciplined, persistent, focused, and driven if you apply the principles in this book and allow yourself to go through the six-step journey. The traits you develop during this journey will change your life in more ways than you can imagine.

Self-discipline will help you follow through with what you need to do to function to the best of your ability. It will help you make consistent and better decisions about the food you eat. It will help you work out regularly and meet your fitness goals. It will help you and remind you to have more fun through the week and throughout your day. Self-discipline will force you to spend your money more wisely and a help you prevent those impulse buys. And most importantly, self-discipline will allow you to live the life that you were designed to live, to help you reach your life vision, and to have fun and be healthy!

Step 6: Celebrate & Refocus - Living Your Ideal Lifestyle

Motivation is what gets you started, and habits are what keep you going. Your rituals are who you are. Step six occurs on numerous occasions during your journey beyond symptoms, and the key to this step is the celebrations. The fourth fundamental of the Core Four is to have fun. If you're not having fun, then what's the point of all of this?

Far too often, as with anything in life, we humans often want something so badly that it's all we think about, but we dread the journey. We want to jump from A to Z yesterday, and we want to conquer our goals tomorrow.

Learn to enjoy the process. Celebrate the small victories, and then move on to the next. Appreciate where you are on the journey, and continue to celebrate the small victories. You know the ultimate destination of where the journey is taking you, so trust that you'll get there and really focus on enjoying each step along the way.

Health knows no age or sex, it doesn't care about your story. Health shows no sympathy and has no feelings. Health listens to no God. There is no age too young or too old, and anyone can play the game. Just know that we have to play the game of health on offense.

Regardless of your current state of health or your current health goals, choosing to make health a significant part of your life can be a ladder to higher levels in your life. Take full responsibility for your health, become super healthy, and you will become an individual with strong character and high value. Build a strong character and be of high value, and you will be generously rewarded in all areas of life.

Mentoring Moment

Game Changer: Your personal journey beyond symptoms will be a rollercoaster ride that you'll never forget. Your journey will be uncomfortable, fun, scary, rewarding, frustrating, and life changing! Luckily for you, you will have developed exceptional rhythms and rituals that have taken your lifestyle to a completely new level.

Six-Steps to Extraordinary Health

Step 1: Mindset – Focus & Make the Decision

Step 2: Motivation – Creating and Achieving Your Health Goals

Step 3: Strategy - Design Your Ideal Lifestyle

Step 4: Accountability - Build a Healthy Environment

Step 5: Take Action – Develop Self-Discipline

Step 6: Celebrate & Refocus – Living Your Ideal Lifestyle

The Core Four – Foundational Principles of Health

1. Function

2. Food

3. Fitness

4. Fun

Own It: To get the most out of this chapter, take the principles that you learned and teach them to someone else. If you can teach them, you will know them. If you know them, you're absolutely going to apply them to your life. Take the time to understand The Journey Beyond Symptoms, and introduce the concept to the people closest to you in your life so that you can begin to build your roadmaps together!

8
Step 1: Mindset
Focus & Make the Decision

"To change your health, you must change your mind."
Ultra Healthy Mindset

M ake the decision to have confidence in your health and freedom from disease. When it comes to your health, there are only two options: one, you are either ready to change your life now, or two, your health is not a priority. How sick does your body have to get before you're willing to make the time and find the resources to make your health a priority? Aside from these two options, everything else is an excuse.

When I was only 21 years old, I made a very uncomfortable decision. I didn't have the time (and I certainly didn't have the money), but for whatever reason, I decided that enough is enough and that I was no longer going to live in my current state of pain. I was tired of suffering and feeling disappointed every time I'd have a flare up and have to change my plans, so I made the time and found the money to change my health. As so often is the case, some people need to hit rock bottom before being able and willing to make The Decision: the decision to make health your number one priority over everything else in your life. I know prioritizing health is a big decision to make, but let's face it, without your health you have nothing. Your relationships suffer, you become a burden to your partner, you're not the parent your kids deserve, you aren't able to reach your professional goals, your money means nothing because you don't have the energy or the will to spend it on fun experiences, and you're simply not the person you were designed to be.

When you're not functioning to the best of your ability or you have a health condition, fulfilling your purpose in life becomes a burden and won't happen at the magnitude you're capable of. So, the first step that you must take, if you're to experience beyond ordinary health, is to make the decision that your health is your greatest asset. Your mindset is the single most important factor in your success. That's why, unlike most diet/weight-loss/fitness/goal setting programs, we focus on helping you create the right mindset from day one rather than building you an overwhelming to-do list and sending you off to fail.

Your Wake-up Call

"Knowing you need to make a change isn't enough.
You have got to find the guts to do it."
Robert Kiyosaki

The first three chapters of this book are your foundation. To the majority of you, the information in those chapters is a complete 180 from everything you thought you knew, were taught, or you read about. This wakeup call isn't meant to be comfortable. You are walking into a battle, as you will be constantly reminded how broken our system is every time you step back out into the real world. People are sick, and sickness is all they know. Everywhere you turn, there will be reminders that there is a pill for every symptom, about how cool it is to drink the sugary drinks, how convenient it is to eat fast food, and how emotional health challenges can be. These challenges are all on purpose; the TV commercials, billboards, magazines, radio, and online advertisements have all mastered the advertising game. In my opinion, all these advertisements give people false hope because the advertisers understand how the brain works. Get a grip, take responsibility, and change your brain.

Mindset is all about how you think. If you change your thoughts, you change your actions. If you change your actions, you change your habits. If you change your habits, you change your life. And if you change your life, you can change the lives of the people around you. That's the purpose of this book, and that's what I do every day in my office: I change people's lives.

In this chapter, I'll lay the groundwork for having the right mindset to be able to work towards experiencing extraordinary health. In addition, I'll help you improve your mindset each and every day by providing resources that will provide you with new insights and perspectives, so you can begin to change what your brain believes to be real.

Health is Emotional

"In order to change, we must be sick
and tired of being sick and tired."
Ultra Healthy Mindset

You are where you are because of who you are and the decisions you have made in your life up until this point. If you are not satisfied or want to improve yourself, then you have to take action. If you want something to change then you are going to have to change. Believe it or not, there are people suffering from health conditions who flat out do not want to get better. They wake up feeling sorry for themselves, accepting their conditions as their new normal, and mosey on through the day with their excuses, complaining to anyone and everyone who is willing to listen. It's true, I see these people every, single day. They truly don't want to get better because if they did, they would have nothing to bitch and gripe about.

The reason these people are like this is because they refuse to make The Decision. They are comfortable with the certainty that they experience on a daily basis, and they fear the unknown of trying to get healthier and having to change. They can't imagine what their lives would be like if they were as healthy as they could be. Worse, they fear what they would have to go through and what they would have to do to reach their health goals. The whole process of getting pushed and pulled in all directions, getting offered advice and recommendations from different doctors, experts, health professionals, and not getting any answers that help or make sense is frustrating, exhausting, and emotionally draining.

The reason health is emotional is because nobody wants to see anyone suffer, especially not the people in our lives who we're close with.

There is an urgent problem in our country where families are being compromised due to misinformation about health, feeling sorry for people who are sick, praying for them, and donating money to support disease research. And we think these are our only options to contribute and help. Let's face it; we can pray, say endless affirmations and have positive thoughts, and give every penny we own to the research labs, and the majority of the sick people are still going to suffer. We need to step up and take action if anything is ever going to change. We need to have a major mind shift in our healthcare system. But since I don't believe that's going to happen anytime soon, the people who are able to break free, make The Decision, and change their mindset towards health are the people who are going to avoid being health statistics.

A good example of this is cancer. Anytime someone is diagnosed with cancer, we can't help but feel for that person's suffering. We must let him or her know that we are here for him and will do anything for him as he gears up for the battle of his life. Well it's no secret that cancer is not something that develops overnight. The truth is that there are hundreds of different forms of cancer. Yet we lump them all under one "Cancer" and throw billions of dollars at this beast as if we're in search of the magic cure.

Now, I understand that since health is emotional and I'm talking about one of the top three killers in America, this information may start to feel uncomfortable to read. However, I'm going to take this information a step further which is going to make the situation even more uncomfortable. I openly do not support cancer research and refuse to donate money to any cancer research program. Most people would consider me a jerk (or insert stronger word here if you're so inclined) because here I am one of the lucky ones who does not suffer from cancer while there are hundreds-of-thousands who are currently suffering and dying. How can someone be so irresponsible and insensitive?

The reality is that I'm more responsible than 98% of the population as I have taken the time to understand how the body works as well as look into these cancer research groups to know where these trillions of dollars are going. As an educated doctor and wellness expert, I assure you there is a better way to spend our healthcare money that would improve the health of our great nation and reduce the rates of cancer, heart disease, and diabetes. The easy thing to do would be to blindly follow the masses and feel sorry for everyone who is suffering, throw money at these foundations, and move on with our busy lives.

So rather than do that, I have dedicated my life to educating people about health so that they become empowered and able to take their own health into their own hands. I have seen thousands of people take the information I have given them and transform their lives – breaking free of their conditions, reaching their health goals, and experiencing the quality of life they could only dream about in the past. I have seen stage IV, terminal cancer patients who were sent home to die go into remission because they decided to do more than just take drugs, pray, and sit there to die as everyone around them felt sorry for them.

Cancer is simply one example on a never ending list. The truth is every disease and/or health condition is made out to be some horrible, unlucky condition that there is no hope for other than the new and improved pill. There are people taking their health back into their own hands every single day, beating health conditions and reaching their health goals without the use of medications, injections, or surgery. Remember that the body is smart, and if we remove any and all interferences and give the body the proper fuel it needs, your body is capable of doing anything.

I'm never worried about the body; I'm usually worried about the brain and mindset – the mind controlling the body usually gets in the way of people reaching their health goals.

The truth is health should be emotional. Health must be emotional. After all, health is our greatest asset. The problem is we tend to tie negative emotions to health the majority of the time. We can empathize and sympathize with those who suffer, but rarely do we celebrate the strong and the healthy. It's like the news; no news is good news, right? We listen to all the negative things that are going on in our country, and we train our brains that all of the stuff we see and hear on a daily basis is normal. And because the negativity is "normal," we accept it and are not even surprised anymore when something crazy happens. Because it's so normal, that crazy "something" happens more and more frequently. That's our healthcare system in a nutshell. Cancer rates have skyrocketed, and heart disease and diabetes are so common that they have become the new normal. So, when someone gets diagnosed, we simply accept the diagnosis, feel sorry for the people with the conditions, and go on with our busy lives, thankful that it wasn't us, at least not this time.

If we continue down this path, our healthcare system will continue to implode as we get sicker and weaker as a nation. If you're going to change your mindset, you need to tie positive emotions to health and escape the dangerous mindset and limiting beliefs that have been created for you. And that's the first step in shifting your mindset. So, decide, do you truly want to be healthy? Why or why not? Do you even feel that you're capable of living a healthy lifestyle? The two things you must do to have a shift in mindset is to develop your WHY and identify your LIMITING BELIEFS, so that you can BE who you need to be, DO what you need to do, and HAVE what you want to have.

Developing Your WHY

> "80% of success is finding a big enough WHY
> and 20% is finding out the HOW."
> **The Pareto Principle**

Why do you want to be healthy? Is it because you don't want to end up like a certain someone in your life who suffered from a health condition? Is it because you want to be there for your spouse, kids, grandkids? Is it so you can best fulfill your life purpose – whatever it may be?

There are no right or wrong answers as to why you want to be healthy just as long you're emotionally tied to your WHY. Your Big Answer has to come from within you. Your WHY has to drive you and push you so that anytime you come across a challenge, any type of resistance, you dig down and you continue pushing forward because your WHY is far more important than any fear or uncertainty that challenges you.

Your WHY has everything to do with you. What do you want out of life? Why do you wake-up in the morning? Why do you do what you do? Quit being so logical and analytical about this. I get it, you work because you need to earn money so that you can provide for your family. I totally get it, and the reality is you could make money doing a thousand other things. My point is just forget everything you think you know and that you think you have to do, and imagine what you would do if money didn't matter. If you find yourself immediately saying, "But money does matter," we have some serious work to do. You see, our brains are not meant to make us happy, they are built to protect us. Our brains are always seeking worst case scenarios – searching for problems.

If you're someone who finds the negative in everything, then this process is going to be a little more difficult but that much more important for you. This difficulty is, in part, due to your having a limiting mindset. And that's okay. The first step is recognizing your limited thinking. If you can be honest with yourself and own up to the fact that you have limiting beliefs, then you're empowered to be able to change your thought pattern. However, as long as your brain is in protective mode, you will always play it safe for fear of failing.

People who fail focus on process, and people who succeed focus on the outcome. Outcome is the big picture. Process is all about the little details which leads to way too many internal conversations. This often leads to anxiety because of anticipation of future events. Right now, as you read this, do you really have any problems? Are there any severe threats around you? Is this book going to jump up and bite you? All is good! Life is good; you're alive and breathing which means you have the opportunity to be and do anything you want. Focus on the now and don't worry about next week or even later today. One day at a time, one hour at a time, one moment at a time!

One of man's greatest fears is failure – not being good enough. If you can embrace this fear, accept this fear, and use it to benefit you, you'll quickly see that failure actually leads to greatness. If we can learn from our mistakes, then we tend to do things better the next time around. So, the problem is not when you fail, the problem is when you quit because you've failed. And do you know what the number one reason for people failing is? They don't have a compelling reason to keep going – a big enough WHY. So, start to think about the WHO or WHAT in your life that makes up your WHY. Who or what is the compelling reason that you are willing to do whatever it takes to get healthy no matter what obstacle stands in your way?

Limiting Beliefs

> "You are the only one who can limit your greatness.
> You don't have to let your past stories define you."
> **Ultra Healthy Mindset**

Our mind has thoughts based on our past experiences. What are the stories that you've been telling yourself that have been holding you back? These are your limiting beliefs. You need to drop these. You need to take 100% responsibility for your thoughts.

To get the results of a healthy person, you need to start thinking like a healthy person and doing what healthy people do. You have to behave like very few people do. Turn off the television, stop gossiping, and start producing. Quit focusing on what's not working, and start focusing on what is working. Don't ever try to solve a problem in a state of stress or anxiety.

Limiting beliefs are thoughts and ideas that you picked up early in life that are simply not true, yet you hold onto them because you don't know any better. You need to get rid of any and all limitations because limiting yourself invalidates your abilities. The reality is this isn't even about you. You need to do this because your WHY is so much bigger than you are.

Because our belief systems are ingrained is us as children, we move through life creating experiences to match our beliefs. Look back at your own life and notice how often you have gone through the same or similar experiences.

If you're suffering from health conditions or symptoms, how do you feel about these conditions? Exhausted? Anxious? Angry? Hopeless? If you stay with that emotion and acknowledge it for a moment, you'll find the limiting belief right beneath the emotion. For example, "exhausted" might be saying, "I've tried anything and everything to no avail, and I'm done living like this." "Anxiety" might be saying, "What will people think of me?" "Anger" might reflect, "Life isn't fair to people like me." Underneath hopelessness might be, "I'm just not meant to be healthy or strong."

Acknowledge that these are beliefs, not truths! This is often the hardest step. Here's the place where choice comes in. Which are you more interested in, defending your limitations to the death or achieving your health goals and desires?

Try on a different belief. Use your imagination and try on a belief that is aligned with what you want. This new belief might be something like, "Even though I've been unhealthy for the majority of my life, I've now learned what to do to be able to turn my lifestyle around so that I can create and then achieve my health goals!"

The trick is to go beyond just saying this belief. You want to really step into this new belief and feel how it feels.

Take different action. This might feel scary, but act as if your new belief is true. In other words, if you really are capable and have learned a tremendous amount from past health conditions, what steps will you take to function at a higher level and become healthier? If you really are the kind of person who eats healthy food, what will you put in your grocery cart?

If you avoid taking any steps based on your new belief, you will just feed your old, limiting belief. Taking action, even the smallest step will help solidify your new un-limiting decision. Your first steps don't have to be perfect, just headed in the right direction. Be sure to acknowledge yourself and celebrate when you've taken that step.

Perhaps you have come across this quote by Marianne Williamson before: "Our deepest fear is not that we are inadequate. Our deepest fear is that we are powerful beyond measure. It is our light, not our darkness that most frightens us. We ask ourselves, 'Who am I to be brilliant, gorgeous, talented, fabulous?' Actually, who are you not to be? You are a child of God. Your playing small does not serve the world. There is nothing enlightened about shrinking so that other people won't feel insecure around you. We are all meant to shine, as children do. We were born to make manifest the glory of God that is within us. It's not just in some of us; it's for everyone. And as we let our own light shine, we unconsciously give other people permission to do the same. As we are liberated from our own fear, our presence automatically liberates others."

Have there been times in your life when you could have made a move toward a better job or a healthier relationship? Or perhaps towards a more challenging, happier existence, and you just didn't? What were you so afraid of? Limiting beliefs may hold you back from taking chances, keep you blind to opportunities in your path, prevent you from accepting gifts offered to you, or simply keep you stuck focusing on the negative aspect of your circumstances.

The most challenging thing with limiting beliefs is that they are often buried deep in our subconscious so that we don't realize they're there, and we can't see what they're doing to us. To discover your own personal, limiting beliefs, you must pay attention to patterns. Honestly, discovering you have a limiting belief is such a huge step forward, if you've gotten there, it's time to celebrate! You know the saying, "knowing is half the battle"? It's really true. When you know and acknowledge your limiting belief as just that — a belief you can choose to change — you are on the right track.

Squash Your ANTs

"When life is sweet, say thank you and celebrate,
when life is bitter, say thank you and grow."
Ultra Healthy Mindset

Before giving you the tools to sharpen your mindset and retrain your brain to a new normal, it is absolutely vital that you address and work towards removing any and all negative thoughts that you routinely get.

Begin by paying attention to how you respond to certain situations. One of my favorite examples is driving a car. Are you the person who is happy-go-lucky and at peace with the wind to your back, or are you the person who is frustrated with how slow the guy in front of you is driving and you're literally yelling at him for cutting you off? Perhaps you're somewhere in between. Regardless, begin to pay attention to how you respond and thoughts that come to mind during different situations throughout the day, and you should be able to get a really good idea if you have good positive thoughts or if you're more on the negative side.

For those of you on the more negative side, you experience what is called Automatic Negative Thoughts or ANTs. You need to start by fighting and getting rid of all of your ANTs. You need to address these thoughts and face them head-on by talking back to your brain, being very straightforward.

A simple, "No thank you, brain, I'm good," will do the trick. As silly as this sounds, talking back is extremely effective. Remember, your brain's number one job is to protect you. Let your brain know that you are okay and no longer in need of certain thoughts. After you begin to get a grip on your thoughts and challenging your brain by talking to yourself, step this process up a notch and let your brain know who is in charge. "I am the master of my thoughts. I determine how I feel. I don't want this negativity, and I refuse to live with it."

I know it may sound or feel awkward to say this to yourself. But what do you have to lose? The biggest challenge you will ever face is having the wrong mindset. Listen, your WHY comes from your heart, and you are emotionally tied to this Big Reason. Your brain is way too logical and will continue to try to interfere and save you from the possibility of failure and fear of the unknown. The hardest journey for anyone is the 18 inches from your brain to your heart. Only your heart knows what you truly want, so the more in tune you become with your body and your feelings, the easier it will be to squash your ANTs and retake control of your limiting mindset.

Automatic Negative Thoughts pop up and flash in your mind without conscious thought. Your brain has been trained and conditioned for years, and your brain believes these thoughts to be normal. Clearly, these are not the thoughts that you want your brain to consider normal.

Negative thinking is a survival strategy that causes us to look for what is wrong so that we can protect ourselves against danger, but all this negative thinking is a very bad strategy because our thoughts actually create reality. So, instead of preventing bad things from happening, we are attracting the bad things into our lives.

Negative thoughts severely limit a person's ability to enjoy his or her life. How you think "moment-to-moment" plays a large role in how you feel - a deep, limbic system function. Negative thoughts can cause you to feel internal discomfort or pain, and they often cause you to behave in ways that alienate you from other people. Hopeful thoughts, on the other hand, influence positive behaviors and lead people to feel good about themselves and be more effective in their day-to-day lives. Hopeful thoughts are also involved in helping people connect with others.

Healing the deep, limbic system requires a person to heal his or her moment-to-moment thought patterns. Unfortunately, there is no formal place where we are taught to ponder our thoughts or to challenge the notions that go through our heads, even though our thoughts are always with us. Most people do not understand how important thoughts are and leave the development of thought patterns to random chance.

Did you know that every thought you have sends electrical signals throughout your brain? Thoughts have actual physical properties. They are real! They have a significant influence on every cell in your body. When your mind is burdened with many negative thoughts, the negativity affects your deep, limbic system and causes deep limbic problems - irritability, moodiness, depression, etc. Teaching yourself to control and direct your thoughts in a positive way is one of the most effective ways to feel better.

There are numerous books and programs available that focus entirely on breaking negative thought patterns. My personal advice is to seek help if you need help. Be willing to work on yourself because you're worth the effort. A positive mindset is a key component in your journey beyond symptoms to extraordinary health as well as in all other aspects of life.

Be – Do – Have

> "The best way to get people to do something
> better is to challenge them."
> **Ultra Healthy Mindset**

As you begin to squash your ANTs, you need to simultaneously feed your brain the fuel it needs to become stronger and more powerful. You can reprogram your brain to have any thoughts that you would like.

Nothing in this world will get you a stronger, clearer, state of mind than starting your day with gratitude. Be thankful and appreciative every single day. Gratitude is not for weirdoes, it's for winners. Successful people are grateful people. Stay away from social media and the news, there is plenty of time in the day to fry your brain. The morning is a time to clear your mind of garbage and power it up with powerful, positive thoughts. Empty out anything negative from the day before, and develop the mindset of a champion. Believe like you will get whatever you can imagine. Say "thank you" in advance for what is already yours. We all have negative emotions and feelings. You have to make a choice. I suggest choosing to not give bitterness, anger, or jealousy valuable space in your mind to poison your life. Instead, be mindful of the thoughts that you allow into your mind.

Our brains are incredibly complex. The RAS – reticular activating system - is a bundle of nerves at our brainstem that takes what you focus on and creates a filter for that focus. The RAS then sifts through the data and presents only the pieces of information that are important to you. So in a way, the RAS seeks information that only validates your beliefs. It filters the world through the parameters you give it, and your beliefs shape those parameters. If you think that you don't stand a chance of experiencing extraordinary health, you probably never will. If you believe that you are disciplined enough to follow your workout program and be fit, you most likely will become fit if you're not already. The RAS helps you see what you want to see and in doing so, influences your actions.

Here's a great example: have you ever bought a car that you absolutely loved and felt it was the perfect, unique car for you only to notice in the first few weeks of driving it that everyone else is driving that same car? That's your reticular activating system at work. And the cool part is you can train your RAS by taking your subconscious thoughts and intertwining them with your conscious thoughts. In other words, if you focus hard on your goals and have great intentions, your RAS will reveal the people, information, and opportunities that will help you achieve them.

For example, if you care about your health, you will become more aware of and seek a healthy lifestyle. If you really want to make exercise an important ritual and become super fit, then set your intent on getting fit and your brain will tune into the right information that helps you do that.

When you look at The Law of Attraction this way, it doesn't seem so "crazy." Simply put: focus on the bad things and you will invite negativity into your life. Focus on the good things, and they will come to you because your brain is seeking them out. This attraction of the positive is not magic, it's your RAS influencing the world you see around you.

Now, here is the problem for most people. Most people think about what they don't want and wonder why the negativity shows up over and over again. For instance, if you are always complaining, the Law of Attraction will bring you more situations to complain about. If you are listening to someone else complain and focusing on that, sympathizing and agreeing with them, you are attracting more situations to yourself to complain about. Your entire life can change by focusing on what you do and want as opposed to what you do not want, what you are afraid of, and what you want to avoid.

One way to master your mind is to learn to quiet your mind. Meditation quiets your mind, helps you control your thoughts, and revitalizes your body. The great news is that you don't have to set aside hours at a time to meditate. Just a few minutes a day can be incredibly powerful for gaining control of your thoughts. To become aware of your thoughts, you can also set the intention, "I am the master of my thoughts." Say this intention often, meditate on it.

Like with any skill, you have a limited natural ability. You have to continuously practice if you wish to better your skill set. If you want to hit the professional level with any skill, that mastery takes commitment, action, and perseverance to be the best.

Mindset is the Fuel – Being before Doing. The idea of "Be – Do – Have" simply implies instead of focusing on what you want to have, focus on who you need to BE and what you need to DO so that you can HAVE what it is that you're after.

Far too often, we find ourselves thinking and living on the Have-Do-Be principle. As a result, we often miss out on our true potentials.

When I finally HAVE _____ (enough money, enough time, enough energy, the perfect body, the perfect house, the perfect car, or a better relationship etc.) then I will DO _____ (work out more, eat cleaner, make my health a priority, spend more time with my family, work less, read more, etc.) and I will BE _____ (healthy, happy, fit, loving, secure, confident, disciplined, etc.).

This backwards thinking is "normal" for the human mind which is why you need to be constantly strengthening your mind. The reality is that you will never HAVE it all. There's always going to be someone or something better, healthier, happier, fitter, better looking, more successful, etc. that you're going to want and be like.

We are all spiritual beings on a human journey. While HAVING serves our human side, HAVING simply doesn't serve our spiritual side nearly as well.

You must BE what you want to be. You must BE healthy in order to DO healthy things in order for you to HAVE a healthy future. You must BE self-disciplined in order to DO certain rhythms and rituals that will allow you to HAVE extraordinary health. You don't attract what you want, you attract what you are.

We've all seen those people who have money and success, but they obviously are not happy. They need more and more and more to try to fill the void of who they are not. They are driven by the HAVE-DO-BE and there's not enough in this world to HAVE before they can BE.

When you choose what you are going to be, you will be challenged in that decision. If you choose to be accountable, you will have lots of opportunities to practice accountability. If you choose to be motivated, you will have lots of opportunities to demonstrate your motivation.

What qualities of other people do you appreciate? Those same qualities reside in you, and you too can claim them. Make the decision, and choose to BE the characteristic's you seek. Realize that you have a choice to make.

Most of us would never feel comfortable going up to somebody and criticizing him right to his face. Yet we criticize ourselves every single day, constantly telling ourselves, "I AM NOT good enough. I am not skinny enough. I am not beautiful enough. I am not smart enough. I'll never be fast enough." Whatever negative self-talk that you have, it's not okay. Do yourself a favor, and zip that up. You have enough things in your life working against you. There is only one you. As long as you are happy and fulfilled, that is truly all that matters in life. As long as you continue to chase pipe dreams and try become someone you were never meant to be, you will never be fully happy or fulfilled.

So, the challenge is to become the success story you were meant to be and show the world what is possible. If you can become that person and do what is necessary, you can assure you will have whatever it is that you're seeking.

Your mindset is the single most important factor that will allow you to live the super-healthy lifestyle that you are capable of. Are you ready to make The Decision? Are you ready to make your health a top priority and to let go of all the excuses that have been keeping you from experiencing the life that you want?

Mentoring Moment

Game Changer: This may quite possibly be the most important chapter in this entire book. Your mindset is absolutely vital and will determine the outcome of your life. Your thoughts are essential to your being and to your health. Because health is emotional, you need to focus on what you truly want to accomplish here, and you have to make The Decision to accomplish what you want. Make The Decision that nothing will get in the way and that you will accomplish what you set out for no matter what.

Make no mistake... this will be an extremely uncomfortable process. It will be challenging, but as you grow and develop into the person you are destined to be, this will also be the most rewarding experience of your life. Change your brain – change your life!

Own It: To get the most out of this chapter, take the principles and the suggested exercises that you learned and teach them to someone else. As you teach them, you will become better versed and aware of your limiting beliefs and ANTs. As you become more aware, you're absolutely going to begin squashing your ANTs and changing your regular thought patterns, ultimately becoming who you need to BE. The upcoming chapters will show you what you need to DO in order to HAVE what you are after.

9

Step 2: Motivation Creating and Achieving Your Health Goals

"Dreams without goals remain dreams and
ultimately fuel disappointment."
Denzel Washington

G oals motivate us to achieve what we desire most, and goals are essential for bettering yourself in any area of life, especially your health. However, with goal setting we face two challenges.

The first challenge you may face is your mindset about goal setting. You've most likely tried setting goals in the past. If you've been successful in achieving the goals you've set, then you enjoy the goal setting process and will enjoy this chapter. However, if you're like most people, you've tried setting goals in the past but have failed to reach your goals. And, if you've done this repeatedly with a lack of results, then you may have a bad taste in your mouth about goal setting that's deterring you or even preventing you from setting more goals.

If you fit into this second group of people, I want to encourage you to not let your past predict your future. In other words, just because you've failed at goal setting in the past does not mean goal setting doesn't work or that goal setting cannot work for you. First, you're not the same person today as you were when you set your previous goals. Give your new self another chance. Second, you may not have been as committed to achieving your goals then as you are today. And third, thinking an activity is impossible just because it hasn't worked yet is illogical. Think about this for a moment...

When you were a child learning to walk, did you give up after falling on your butt dozens, maybe even hundreds of times? Of course not. The fact that you're walking today proves that you didn't throw in the towel and stop trying. You got up and tried again. And when you fell, you may have whined or cried a bit... but then you tried again and again until you walked.

Goal setting does work. And if you're serious about achieving extraordinary health – which I think you are based on the fact you've read this far – then I want to encourage you to forget your past failures and work through this chapter with an open mind and an open heart. You can set and achieve your goals.

The second challenge you may face is what I call "fear-based thinking." Fear-based thinking is knowing what you don't want and basing your goals and your intents on your fears, not your desires. As we learned in the previous chapter, what you think about is usually what you get. So, by focusing on what you don't want, you can attract what you fear instead of achieving what you desire.

In addition, knowing that you don't want to end up unhealthy like your parents or experience sickness like a good friend from your childhood does not motivate you to take action. Instead, we want to set goals that inspire you and motivate you to act and achieve.

So, how are you going to face these challenges head on and achieve your health goals? In just a moment, I'm going to walk you through three exercises to help you create and achieve your goals. But first, I want to give you some important tips for creating your health goals.

Tips for Creating and Achieving Your Goals

There are three important points I want you to remember when setting your goals:

1. Focus on what you want, not what you don't want.

2. Be bold but realistic.

3. There is power in writing down your goals.

First, like I mentioned earlier, fear-based thinking can be a big challenge for some people. If you really want to achieve your health goals, I encourage you to focus on what you want.

For example, if you want to "eliminate back pain" (a fear-based goal), consider refocusing your intent on making your "back and core strong and healthy" (a desire-based goal). Remember, your brain finds a way to achieve what you want. So, if you tell your brain to eliminate back pain, then your brain will find ways to keep your body and your back in pain.

It's just like telling yourself "don't think of the color red." What does your brain immediately think of? Red. The same is true for your goals. Keep your goals and your intent focused on what you want.

Next, I want you to be bold but realistic. I know that may sound contradictory, so let me explain. I want you to be bold, and set goals that inspire you. I don't want you to limit yourself on what you can achieve. If you can envision a goal, I believe you can achieve the goal.

However, while I want you to be bold, I also want you to be realistic with your goals. For example, if you weigh 200 pounds now and you want to trim down to a slim, 180 pounds (notice that I didn't say "lose 20 pounds"), setting the goal to do so in a week is unrealistic (and not healthy). So, to make this goal bold yet realistic, set the goal for one month from today. That way you have four weeks to trim down to 180 pounds (five pounds per week).

Lastly, there is power in writing down your goals. The reason is because when you write down a goal, you subconsciously commit yourself to achieving that goal. That's why all successful people write down their goals. They know that once the goal is articulated and written down, they have no choice but to "go all-in" and make the goal a reality.

In addition to these points while setting goals, there are two more tips I want you to keep in mind while you're going through the process of achieving your goals. And those two tips are:

1. Don't let anyone dissuade you from going after what you want.

2. Failing to achieve a goal does not make you a failure.

The unfortunate truth is the majority of the population doesn't want the best for you, because your pushing forward to be better reflects poorly on their choices. So, if you tell other people about your goals and your intentions, you will have pushback. This pushback doesn't mean that the people you tell (family, friends, etc.) don't love you. But they'll give you their opinions based on their past failures.

Do you remember when I said, "don't let your past predict your future"? Well, the same holds true for other people in your life. You can't let other people's past failures predict your future. Your goals are your goals, not their goals. So, their opinion as to whether you can accomplish your goals is irrelevant and unfounded.

My recommendation is to be selective with who you share your goals with. You don't need other peoples' negativity in your head messing with your mindset. To achieve your goals, you'll need focused, positive energy.

The two people who need to know about your health goals are your health coach and your significant other. Your health coach (if you have one) will help you set up goals anyway. He or she can be trusted to push you and support you. Telling your significant other, on the other hand, depends on whether he or she is supportive or not. If he is not supportive of your goals, then I'd forgo telling him. However, if he is supportive and wants the best for you (which is most likely the case), then tell him what you're committed to achieving and what help you'd like from him. A supportive partner can be instrumental in helping you achieve your desires.

The last point I want to make before we move into the goal-setting section is the fact that failing to achieve a goal does not make you a failure. The only time we fail in life is when we give up. We're human so messing up in some way at some point is inevitable. What really matters is that we don't give up or give in. If you miss a workout, then brush off the lapse and recommit to exercising the next day.

If you slip up and eat something that's not good for you, then recommit to eating better moving forward. Mistakes and mishaps are not the end of the world. They are tests. Not the kind of test where you're graded or that you either pass or fail. Instead, they are tests to determine who you are. Are you a quitter or are you a fighter?

Keep that question in mind as you continue reading and as you fight for what you want in your life. My bet is that you're a fighter, and you're the type of person who will achieve your goals no matter what or who gets in your way!

With that all that said, let's start setting and achieving your goals and desires.

What's Your Vision for Your Future?

"A man without a vision for his future
always returns to his past."
Ultra Healthy Mindset

I believe the act of setting goals is bigger than just achieving goal after goal. I believe that goal setting, at its core, is about becoming a better version of you. Yes, in just a moment, we'll set 3-month and 12-month goals, so you can have a target to aim for. But first, we need to look at who you want to become 30 years from now. By doing so, we can work backwards, and you can become that person one day at a time.

To help you begin this process, let's imagine two scenarios:

First, if you could fast forward 30 years from now, would you want to be as healthy and experiencing the same quality of life as your parents currently are?

If your parents are healthy and living a great life, then I suggest you use your parents as role models and seek guidance as to what you can do to assure that happens. Their state of health didn't happen by accident. Take time to model after their actions, so you too can live life like they are.

Now, I don't know what you're parents' current state of health is, but the facts state that the majority of us have parents who are unhealthy and struggling. If that describes your parents, then it's important that you think through this:

Do you believe when your parents were your age that they hoped they would end up the way that they are now?

Of course, they didn't! Very few people take the time to think ahead and put together a game plan for what they're ultimately after. Most people simply go where life takes them and wake up one day wondering how they got to where they are and in the condition they're in.

I don't want that for you and I would imagine neither do you! That's why I'm going to help you create a 30-year goal... Your Vision... so you can look into the future and make better choices today to live the future you deserve.

Now, let's travel ahead in time to the future and imagine another scenario:

Picture yourself as an old man or woman sitting on your front porch in a rocking chair. What are you thinking about? Do you have any regrets?

Listen, I strongly believe that when that day comes, you won't be remembering or thinking about your failures, you'll be thinking about the things that you didn't do and that you wish you had: the "should'ves" and the "would'ves" of our life.

But I'm here to tell you that you don't have to have any regrets. You can live life to the fullest and enjoy every moment... if you plan ahead now so you can live a healthy and fulfilling life. Yes, life is going to be a rollercoaster of a journey, but you can do anything and everything you desire if you want it bad enough.

Now, to help you become clear on what you envision your future to be, take a moment and answer several questions:

1. How do I see myself 30 years from now? _____

_____

_____

2. What does my life look like 30 years from now? _____

_____

_____

3. What am I doing 30 years from now? _____

_____

_____

4. Who am I enjoying life with 30 years from now? _____

_____

_____

5. How do I look and feel 30 years from now? _____

_____

_____

To give you an example, here's how I initially answered these questions: health is a top priority of mine. I am fit well into my retirement years. I have access to all the personal equipment I need to keep active and keep in tip-top shape. I have a regular routine I follow with an awesome top-notch team of health experts who keep me functioning to the best of my ability. My wife and I continue to eat super clean and enjoy the exotic flavors of power foods. I have more energy than I have ever experienced in my life and I am more productive now than ever before. My kids are impressed with my well-being, and my grandkids beg to spend weekends away with us! Traveling the world with my wife and enjoying each other's company has never been so pleasurable and enjoyable! Life is amazing, and I have zero regrets. I love my lifestyle, and I am grateful that I made the decision to live this way 30 years ago.

Take some time now to answer these five questions. Your answers will set the tone for the rest of this chapter and the rest of your life.

But 30 Years Is So Far Away

I know that 30 years seems so far away. But it's not. The next 30 years is going to fly by faster than we'd like. And if we don't look ahead and determine the person we want to become, then we may find ourselves 30 years older and not living the life we want.

I don't want that for you. And I know that you don't want that for yourself. So, if you feel like you're getting stuck trying to answer these questions, this resistance is probably for one of two reasons.

First, if you're getting stuck, you may be thinking too hard. To be able to answer these questions you must avoid using your "educated brain," and instead, listen to your body and your heart. The answers aren't always logical. The answers should be emotional. You should feel the answers in your gut. So, if you're getting stuck, attempt to let go of logic and feel your answers.

Second, you may feel that making these decisions today sets the future in stone. Please understand that your 30-year health goals can change. In fact, they will change as your life-vision changes and as you see what you're capable of achieving. For now, determining the type of person you want to become is important, so you can start your new journey on the right foot.

One Day at a Time

You may be wondering, "How on earth am I ever going to reach my 30-year health goals?" The answer is one day at a time. You see, every decision you make either takes you closer to or farther away from the person you want to become. That's why your identity (who you want to become) is so important because your core values will guide every decision you make in your life and for your health.

Far too often when people are faced with challenging decisions, they are tempted to opt for what will bring them short-term gratification. However, the issue with the short-term gratification is that it typically leads to long-term pain. For example, smoking a cigarette, drinking a soda, eating fast food, hitting the snooze button, skipping a workout, and taking medication for a symptom may feel good and provide some people with short-term gratification. After all, none of these examples would kill you if you decided to do any of them today.

But here's the problem with that type of thinking: because you have no immediate, negative consequences partaking in any of these actions today, you give your subconscious brain permission to partake in the same, detrimental actions again tomorrow. These actions may seem harmless now, but the decision to feel short-term gratification today with one of these unhealthy actions starts a vicious cycle that can continue the rest of your life and impact your health long-term. And the longer the cycle continues, the longer breaking these bad habits or reversing any negative effects will take (if you can reverse the negative effects at all!).

Like it or not... the actions you take today determine your actions tomorrow. Real success comes when we can deal with the small inconveniences today, so we can experience long-term results for the rest of our days.

Creating and Achieving Your Health Goals

Now that you have a better vision for the future and you know who you want to be and how you want to live in 30 years, let's take that overall vision and work backwards to make your vision a reality.

How? First, we're going to start by setting three, 12-month goals (or annual goals). That way you have a target to focus on for the next year. You see, your 30-year goals give you a vision for who you want to be in the future. But those goals are too far into the future and too broad for your brain to target and hit.

That's why we're going take your 30-year goals and move toward your vision with what we can realistically accomplish over the next twelve months.

Then, we're going to set three, 3-month goals (or quarterly goals) based on your annual goals. Doing so allows us to take a big, 12-month goal and break it down into a manageable, easier goal to hit.

Look, most people fall into the "New Year's Resolution" mindset trap. They see goals in big blocks of time (i.e. one year), and they ask themselves "what am I going to do this year?" While that's a good start (and should be done), grouping goals in one-year chunks makes reaching those goals more difficult. Why? Because just like eating processed, sugar-laden food today has no immediate, negative consequences that you can see or feel, eating a diet chalk-full of organic whole foods today has no immediate, positive benefits that you can see or feel. And not seeing progress dissuades the best of us from being persistent and sticking with our long-term goals.

I'm not going to allow you to fall into this mindset trap. Instead, we're going to set 12-month goals (long-term goals) that will help you move toward your 30-year vision, and then we're going to break those annual goals into manageable 3-month goals (short-term goals) that get you excited and are easier to achieve.

Application Exercise #5

With your 30-year vision in mind, what do you want to accomplish over the next twelve months? Do you want to remove all excess sugar from your diet and only eat nutrient-dense, whole foods? Do you want to lose 50 pounds and get into better shape? Do you want to run a half marathon or participate in some other type of race or event? Do you want to eliminate the need for medication? Do you want to address your digestion issues (constipation, stomach pains, etc.)? Do you want to stop experiencing the pain and suffering of having migraines?

If you knew you couldn't fail, what would you like to accomplish over the next year? In the space provided, write down three, 12 -month goals. Remember to focus on what you want and be bold but realistic. (You can download the "Creating Then Achieving Your 30-Year Health Goals" worksheet at InspiredToBeHealthy.com)

1. _____

_____

2. _____

_____

3. _____

_____

Excellent! Next, I'd like you to use the space provided and write down your reasons for wanting to achieve these three goals. For example, if one of your 12-month goals is to trim down from 230 pounds to 180 pounds (i.e. lose 50 pounds), why do you want to lose the weight and trim down? Do you want to lose the weight so you can lower your risk of heart disease and diabetes? Do you want to trim down, so you can eliminate the spare tire around your mid-section? Do you want to get in better shape, so you can look better in a bathing suit or so your signifi-cant other looks at you like she used to?

Your reasons are your reasons, so make them personal and emotional. The more personal and emotional you make your reasons, the more motivation you'll have for achieving them.

Write down your personal and emotional reasons here...

1. _____

_____

2. _____

_____

3. _____

_____

Terrific! Now that you have your 12-month goals and you've written down the reasons you want to accomplish those goals, let's break down your annual goals into quarterly goals. That way you can systematically achieve your long-term goals with-out getting overwhelmed or losing your motivation.

So, look at each of your 12-month goals and think about what the first stepping stone is for you to achieve your long-term goals. For example, if one of your 12-month goals is to trim down from 230 pounds to 180 pounds (i.e. lose 50 pounds), I'd divide 50 pounds by 52 weeks in a year to figure out how much weight I need to lose each week.

In this example, I'd have to lose (roughly) one pound each week to achieve my goal. Very doable, right? Since there are twelve to thirteen weeks in three months, my first 3-month goal would be to lose twelve to thirteen pounds in the next three months. And since we want to focus on what we want, I'd rephrase that goal to sound like this: "I will safely trim down from 230 pounds to 218 pounds by [DATE] and enjoy the process of becoming healthier."

If another 12-month goal of yours is to remove all excess sugar from your diet, then I'd look at what your diet looks like today and figure out what you can "substitute" for the excess, sugary foods. For example, if you drink one to three sodas a day, then a great 3-month goal is to replace the soda with water instead. Not only will this goal be easier than eliminating all excess sugar from your diet right away, this "stepping-stone goal" will allow you to take a big step forward so you can build some much-needed momentum.

In the space provided, write down three, 3-month goals that correspond to your three, 12-month goals:

1. _____

_____

2. _____

_____

3. _____

_____

Again, the more personal and emotional your goals, the more motivation you'll have for achieving them. So, take a moment now and write down your personal and emotional reasons for wanting to achieve your three-month goals...

1. _____

_____

2. _____

_____

3. _____

_____

I cannot stress this enough... your reason(s) for wanting to achieve your goals is vital for motivating you to stick with your goals when times get hard. For instance, trimming down from 230 pounds to 180 pounds isn't very motivating by itself. But, if you want to trim down so you can lose your spare tire and have your significant other look at you with his or her bedroom eyes again, then that changes everything. Instead of trying to lose weight, you're now transforming your body to increase your significant other's libido or to save your dying marriage before it's too late. Do you see the difference?

Lastly, I want you to remember that your 3-month and 12-month goals are smaller steps along your path to achieving to your 30-year vision. If you can set a strong enough goal now to push you and motivate you, then you will begin to see positive change in your life. And that little bit of change will motivate you just enough to keep pushing forward and seeing a little more change. And that additional change will motivate you even more, so you keep moving forward and see more change.

As you continue to push forward you will begin to develop habits. And if you develop good, consistent habits and rhythms in your life, then you'll soon be living a healthy lifestyle!

Mentoring Moment

Game Changer: Your health goals are the vital component that is going to motivate you to begin your journey beyond symptoms. If you can get over the hump of setting strong, powerful health goals and get started, the roadmap we are about to create will guide your first, baby steps in the right direction. Commit to completing the Application Exercise and forget about trying to figure out how you're going to achieve these goals – dream big and get your goals down on paper.

Own It: To get the most out of this chapter, take the principles that you learned and teach them to someone else. If you can teach them, you will know them. If you know them, you'll apply them to your life and achieve the goals you desire most.

10
Step 3: Strategy
Design Your Ideal Lifestyle

"How you do anything is how you do everything."
T. Harv Eker

With our Healthcare system exposed, the definition of health established, your 30-year vision, 12-month goals and 3-month goals set, the next step is to create your roadmap and decide which route will best lead you to your goals.

The Core Four

Your Roadmap will consist of four, core principles of health which we will refer to as the "Core Four." In order for you to be able to achieve your 30-year health goals, you will be required to be strong in all four of these principles. You will be able to focus on as few as one of these principles in order to achieve your 3-month goals, but we will slowly introduce the entire Core Four while working to achieve your 12-month goals.

The Core Four Principles of Health are simply the breakdown of your lifestyle. They are as follows:

1. Function

2. Food

3. Fitness

4. Fun

There's no one single principle that has the capability to make you as healthy as you would like to be. There is no quick fix or shortcuts when it comes to experiencing extraordinary health. The reason health conditions are so common here in America is because we have allowed the definition of health to evolve into something more convenient, something that takes the responsibility out of the people's hands and something that can be "fixed" easily. Health is not something that can be "fixed," health is a lifestyle and a way of life.

Your health is your greatest asset. Once you lose it, health is often tough and even sometimes impossible to get back, and you could find yourself left with nothing. Let's review The Core Four Principles of Health so that you can begin to familiarize yourself with them and what reaching your 30-year health goals and experiencing extraordinary health will realistically take. As you read through these four principles, begin to pay attention to where you may need to shift your focus once you begin working towards your 3-month goals.

1. Function (Brain-Spine-Body Connection)

"Each person carries their very own doctor inside of themselves. Far too often, people are unknowing of this truth. The patient is at their best when they give the doctor who resides within themselves a chance to go to work."

Albert Schweitzer, Nobel Prize Winner

The first of the Core Four Principles of Health is "function." This should not come as a surprise to you as we learned in the first two chapters that the definition of health is the optimal function of your body. So of course, function is going to be the key factor to reaching your health goals. You also learned that there is a huge difference between being fit and being healthy. Fitness plays a vital role in overall health. However, you simply cannot achieve extraordinary health if you are not functioning at the best of your ability.

If your body is functioning optimally, then it is working the way it was designed to – with zero interference. As a reminder, the brain controls every single function of the body. The brain does this by sending life energy down through your spinal cord and out hundreds and thousands of nerves to the vital organs, muscles, glands, tissue and cells in your body.

Knowing this piece of information, incorporating a strategy or system that will strengthen, protect, remove, and avoid any interference to your brain, spinal cord, and the rest of your nervous system is vital. There are several ways you can go about doing this. Below are my top four recommendations that I believe everyone in the world should take advantage of:

1.1 Corrective Care Chiropractic Adjustments

1.2 Functional Neurology

1.3 Spinal Hygiene

1.4 Stress Reduction

1.1 Corrective Care Chiropractic Adjustments

"The power that made the body heals the body."
BJ Palmer

There is a false premise in America that chiropractic is for neck pain and back pain. This is the furthest thing from the truth. In fact, chiropractic has nothing to do with neck pain and back pain, and chiropractic has everything to do with your nervous system and how well you function. You see, chiropractors are experts of the spine, similar to the way that dentists work with teeth and cardiologists with the heart.

The reason that a chiropractor focuses on the spine is because the spine has two functions. First, the spine supports you and holds you upright. This is called your posture. Second, the spine protects your spinal cord. A healthy spinal cord is essential to your overall health. Making sure that your spine is doing its job and protecting your spinal cord perfectly is extremely important.

Because stress attacks the weakest part of the body, understanding exactly where you are weak and where you carry your stress is also very important. A Chiropractor is the best doctor to detect weaknesses and vulnerabilities in the spine and, therefore, in the human body.

These doctors can tell a lot about someone's health based on his or her posture. If you have poor posture (uneven shoulders, hunched back, rotated pelvis, a head tilt, etc.) there is a strong chance that you have postural distortions and shifts that are causing physical stress on your spinal cord and nerves. If you are at least aware of your weaknesses and vulnerabilities, you can strengthen those areas, break bad habits, and teach your body a new normal so you can be strong and healthy in those areas of your body. This will allow you to handle stress better and age more gracefully than someone who has a weak posture that is progressively worsening over time.

Long story short, get your spine checked. This is a must for everyone. The tricky part will be finding a good Corrective Care Chiropractor who doesn't simply limit himself to treating back pain. He or she must be experts at understanding how the body works and how every single person is uniquely different.

Unfortunately, over 90% of chiropractors believe that chiropractic has to do with neck pain and back pain. They think this way because that's how insurance companies tell them to think. Does chiropractic help with neck pain and back pain? Of course, it does, but I assure you that you are not going to die from neck or back pain. What will catch up to you is simply treating symptoms and ignoring the underlying cause of those symptoms because those irritated nerves that you're feeling will progressively worsen. At that point, the organs that those nerves innervate have been working overtime, and now that there's pressure on the nerves, those organs are ready to shut down entirely and send your body into a state of dis-ease. Don't let this happen.

Instead, you want to find a Corrective Care Chiropractor. No, he won't be "in-network" with your insurance because he will not stoop down and tell you what the insurance companies want him to tell you. He'll be honest with you and tell you what you NEED to hear as opposed to what you would LIKE to hear. Make no mistake: this will be the best investment you make in your health. Period. End of story!

I assure you will learn more about your body during your initial checkup than you have in your entire life. That's my guarantee to you. If you take the information he gives you and run with it, the initial checkup will allow you to function at a level that you haven't experienced in years. Some of you will function better than you have in your entire lives.

I personally choose to proactively incorporate Corrective Care Chiropractic adjustments as part of my roadmap to hit my own, personal 30-year health goals. I get adjusted and have my kids adjusted once a week, at minimum. I would strongly encourage you to do the same because I assure you that there is no better strategy to ensure you function to the best of your abilities.

1.2 Functional Neurology

"The energy or active exercise of the mind constitutes life."
Aristotle

Traditionally, neurology tends to look at the disease of the nervous system as black-and-white with one side being optimal neurologic function and the other being neurological disease such as tumors, strokes etc. By now, you're aware that our healthcare system takes a reactive approach towards health. Rather than waiting until your body breaks down and you have to see a neurologist for a condition you are suffering from, be proactive and see a functional neurologist on a regular basis.

Modern research has shown that brain function can be dramatically improved in a way that was once considered impossible. Functional Neurology uses specifically designed therapies to enhance the performance of your brain and nervous system. This unique approach offers new hope for people suffering from a wide variety of conditions, and more importantly, these techniques can be used proactively.

Through careful assessment, a Functional Neurologist can not only determine which areas of a person's nervous system are weak but also devise an appropriate treatment to improve the quality of how his or her nervous system functions. The man often credited with the origin of this premise is Dr. Ted Carrick, who has been researching and teaching this model since the mid-1970s.

It's been my experience that the Functional Neurologists who avoid medicine all together tend to be the more creative and successful at improving the quality of life of their patients. I personally choose to proactively use functional neurology as part of my roadmap and have monthly appointments scheduled out as a rhythm and ritual of my life. I would strongly encourage you to do the same.

1.3 Spinal Hygiene

The vast majority know to practice Oral Hygiene by brushing our teeth every day. We all know to practice Cleansing Hygiene by showering every day. The minute I bring up Spinal Hygiene, people look at me like I'm the weird one. We'll pay thousands of dollars to have our children's teeth straightened because God forbid we send our kids to school with crooked teeth. But when it comes to addressing a child's poor posture and crooked spine, that thing that protects your child's life-line (their spinal cord), we put spinal health on the back burner as if it's no big deal. Priorities NEED to change here!

Spinal Hygiene helps you preserve your spine, the structure that supports your posture and protects your spinal cord and is essential to your overall health. Spinal Hygiene exercises should be done daily and become part of your daily routine, like brushing your teeth and taking a shower. Spinal Hygiene exercises include strengthening posture, restoration of normal spinal curvatures, range of motion exercises, and retraining the muscle-memory connection of the muscles that attach to the individual bones that make up your spine.

I personally perform my spinal hygiene exercises every day by dedicating ten to twenty minutes after my morning workouts to ensure that I practice spinal hygiene regularly. I strongly encourage you incorporate spinal hygiene into your daily rhythms as soon as you see a Corrective Care Chiropractor and find out where you have weak and vulnerable postural distortions. Correct those areas and strengthen them as quickly as possible, and you will handle stress better than you ever have in your life!

1.4 Stress Reduction

"Stress Attacks the Weakest part of the Body."
Ultra Healthy Mindset

How can one experience a stress-free life? The answer is you can't.

You can reduce stress, minimize it, and even better handle it, but there's no avoiding stress all together. When you fully understand how stress attacks the weakest part of the body – see chapter six – you immediately acknowledge the need to strengthen any and all vulnerabilities in your body.

There are a ton of techniques out there that will allow you to minimize your stress and temporarily handle stress better. However, unless you're going to do yoga, breathing exercises, meditation, etc. twenty-four hours a day, seven days a week, you will be impacted by stress.

The answer to combatting everyday stress in your life is to minimize it to the best of your abilities. This requires having an empowering morning ritual. You are the most important person in your life. Take care of yourself first thing in the morning then spend the rest of the day caring for others. Take care of yourself by strengthening your mind and by taking care of yourself physically - by fueling your body with appropriate nutrients and getting your workout in. Don't fall into the reactive mind-set: hitting the snooze button, checking social media, or watching the news while stuffing your face with an unhealthy breakfast.

I personally start my days off with positive thoughts and good energy as opposed to stressed out and anxiety-ridden thinking about all that has to get done. Getting up two hours before you have any scheduled event is a good strategy that will allow for you to avoid the craziness of a rushed morning. If you can start your day off in a controlled, empowered fashion, you're more likely to be in control of your day and avoid the unexpected stressors.

2. Food

"Sometimes I think our ancestors would laugh through their tears if they could see how we eat. We eat mostly from colorful boxes and cans. We spray our vegetables and fruits with deadly chemicals, then ship them half-way around the world before we eat them. It's been a grand experiment in the wonders of technology, but what a price we're paying in our health! Many scientific experiments have now demonstrated that if we simply return to eating more traditional, natural foods, the body often begins to heal itself. And, it's becoming impossible to heal personal symptoms, unless they are understood in relationship to the need to heal the planet."

Kristina Turner, *The Self-Healing Cookbook*

When it comes to food, answer this simple question. Why do you eat?

To the majority of Americans, eating is a past time. We've made eating out regularly socially acceptable as a good way to catch up with friends, family, and loved ones. While we're out, we eat massive portions of food, often three times larger than we really need, and after that we pile down a sugar bomb of a dessert. And on top of that, we wash all that food down with a giant soda pop or some other sugary toxic beverage. There's absolutely no reason or validity behind any of this other than we've made over-eating the social norm.

If we're not eating out, we're usually eating because we're bored. If you surround yourself with junk food, don't be surprised when you eat it. You are setting yourself up to eat poorly.

The real reason we are supposed to eat is to fuel our bodies, give our bodies the nutrients needed for optimal function, and to eliminate toxins to enhance our youth and vitality.

Speaking of toxins, our food habits are one of the biggest stressors we put on our bodies. Right next to the over-medicating problem we have here in America, the toxins and chemicals we consume in our foods are the largest chemical stress we endure.

Food can be complicated. Everywhere you turn there's a new trend or fad diet offering false hope and empty promises. However, there is no magic diet that if you do it for 10, 30, or 60 days you will be magically healthy. If you would like to experience extraordinary health, you need to change your food habits. You need to eat good, clean, healthy food, and eat these foods regularly and often. This needs to be your lifestyle, not just a temporary diet program you're trying out for a few weeks. Eating healthy is a lifestyle, not a temporary fad.

Here are the top three strategies that will allow you to take baby steps and incorporate changes that will lead to your new healthy lifelong diet:

2.1) Consume Water

2.2) Eat Real Food

2.3) Incorporate Supplementation

2.1 Consume Water

"Thousands have lived without love, not one without water."
W. H. Auden

Introducing water is the easiest and most effective way to see an immediate impact on your health. The majority of Americans are dehydrated on a daily basis, and most are unaware of their own dehydration. Begin to consume less caffeinated and sugary drinks throughout the day, and replace them with water. Eventually water will be your beverage of choice, and you'll learn that there's really no need to drink anything other than water.

A simple strategy is to drink water first thing in the morning before you do anything else. Drinking water in the morning has countless benefits, such as firing up your metabolism, flushing out toxins, fueling your brain and body, and hydrating you for the entire day. I personally drink 32oz. of water in the first hour that I'm awake and another 32oz. in the next two hours of the day. And then throughout the day, I always have a water bottle with me.

If you don't like the taste of water, then I suggest mixing your water with a splash of organic lemon juice or lime juice to change up the taste. In addition, and this may not be the answer you were looking for, your body needs water to exist, so give yourself plenty of water and learn to enjoy water whether you like the taste or not.

What kind of water should you drink? With all types of "water" on the market today, people sometimes get confused as to what kind of water is best. Should you drink straight from the tap? Should you drink spring water in bottles? I could go on but let me make this simple for you. I would highly suggest incorporating a water filtration system for your entire household. The metals and the toxins in typical, city water are rather disturbing. And the sad part is most people can't taste the metals because they're so used to the taste. Listen, if you drink filtered water long enough and then attempt to drink city water straight from the sink, you will wonder how you ever drank that contaminated water in the first place. It's that bad!

Plus, this water is not good for you to drink or use to shower. You see, your skin is your body's largest organ, and anything that touches your skin can and will be absorbed into your body. Long term, this exposure will have negative effects. That's why I highly recommend that everyone invests in a water filtration system for their homes. The few thousand dollars these systems cost you will be one of the best investments you can make into your overall health.

2.2 Eat Real Food

"It's bizarre that the produce manager is more important to my children's health than the pediatrician."
Meryl Streep

The key to giving your body the nutrients it needs for optimal function is to eat real food. In the perfect world, you would minimize sugar, wheat, and dairy, or eliminate these foods all together. In addition, you would consume organic and non-GMO foods. I will encourage you to take baby steps and achieve the lifestyle of eating real food and fueling your body with only the best fuel for you to function at your best.

A simple example would be to put together a veggie bowl in the morning and take the veggies with you for the day. I promise you, when you are sitting around bored and find yourself reaching for the typical snack, the veggie bowl will more than suffice. If you put a bowl of greasy potato chips in front of you, those chips will be gone by day's end. The same goes for a plateful of cookies. However, you may be surprised to find out the same goes for a bowl of veggies.

Another simple hack that you can start doing tomorrow is making a smoothie in the mornings. We all know that breakfast is the most important meal of the day, however, the majority of Americans break their overnight fast by consuming a bowl full of sugar in the form of cereal. This is not the way to fuel your high-powered body. If you can get into the rhythm of making a smoothie as part of your breakfast, you will be less likely to fill up on empty foods.

NOTE: Fruit-based smoothies are better than the sugary, processed cereals that the majority of Americans consume; however, since you ideally want to eat a 3:1 ratio of veggies to fruit during the day, I recommend finding some good smoothies you can make using both veggies and fruit. These types of smoothies are better for you and will give you the energy you to need between meals.

Now, if you're willing to take the small amount of time to make your morning smoothie and your veggie bowl for the day, you might as well take another tiny step and set aside some time for meal planning and food prep. This tiny step is especially important for your lunches since the majority of Americans are away from home during the lunch hour. If you plan ahead of time and bring a lunch with you, it's going to be easier to avoid going out for lunch or grabbing the quick convenient foods at the local gas station. Meal planning and food prep is something that takes time and a bit of practice, but I assure you that meal prep is a skill worth learning. A habit of food planning and meal prepping will surely lead you towards your 30-year health goals.

When you're trying to switch over to eating real foods, simply don't buy fake foods. Avoid buying processed foods and sugary drinks, and you won't be able to consume them at home. Avoiding fake foods really is that easy. If you buy them (even with the intention that you're not going to consume them) you will most certainly consume them. Quit impulse buying at the grocery store, and begin to limit and eventually eliminate all together processed and convenient foods. Instead, eat fresh foods that will supply value to your health goals.

Now that you know what to buy, begin experimenting with meal planning. Create a list of what you intend to eat for the week by planning out your meals. Build your grocery list with intention and purpose, so when you're at the grocery store, you're on a mission rather than a food-buying adventure. Experiment with this process because that's what this process is; you'll learn rather quickly what you need to get through a week of smoothies, veggie bowls, lunches, and dinners. As long as you get in the habit of planning for success, you will succeed. Plans rarely fail you. Our failing is that we fail to plan. Take into consideration your entire family during this process. Kids can and will only eat what's in the house, so quit giving them excuses to eat unhealthy!

If food is an area that you know you struggle with and the idea of eating real food and eliminating garbage from your diet is overwhelming, my recommendation is to take the baby steps mentioned above. When you begin to develop some good habits with eating real food, consider partaking in a purification program. A proper program will lead you to eating whole foods and eliminating sugar, wheat, and dairy from your diet. The program that I personally use twice a year is a 21-day program designed to purify your body, cleanse your liver and gut, and develop some strong eating habits that incorporate organic, non-GMO, real foods. This program will also help you get in the mindset for meal planning as well as food prep. Eating healthy takes time and energy, but you're totally worth it!

2.3 Incorporate Supplementation

"If you can't eat it, take it."
Ultra Healthy Mindset

Taking supplements is an effective way of supplying your body the extra support and fuel that your body needs to experience extraordinary health. Getting all the nutrients and benefits your body deserves directly from food is nearly impossible. The key to using supplements is to use them as they are designed to be used - to supplement a good nutritional diet. Far too often, people use supplements like drugs in the hopes to get a quick, immediate fix to a problem they have been putting up with for years.

When considering supplementations, I personally recommend you take good-quality, whole-food supplements or avoid them all together. Buying and using generic vitamins out of the buy-one-get-one-free bin from your major retailers is not going to do the trick. In fact, not only are you wasting your money, you're causing chemical stress to your body from all the fillers and man-made ingredients used in them. You would literally be better off not taking anything than shoving these into your body.

There are several premium, whole-food supplement companies in the market, and as long as you're consuming whole-food based products, any of the brands will benefit you. "Whole food" simply means that the supplements are entirely comprised of food-based ingredients with no additives or fillers. You get the benefits of eating real foods without having to eat the massive amount of food required to get the same nutritional value that the supplements provide. To take this concept a step further and help you fully understand this concept, many of the ingredients come from the roots of certain plants. So rather than eating 50 carrots or ten heads of broccoli (obviously not an easy task), there are supplements that will provide a similar nutritional value and will be a lot easier on your tummy and your digestive system!

My recommendation is that you find a naturopath doctor or other medical professional who specializes in whole-food supplements as there are hundreds of products and finding good-quality supplements can be overwhelming for the average consumer. In addition, those who specialize in these types of supplements have several tools and systems they can utilize to pinpoint where your body needs assistance or which products will get you functioning at an overall higher level. As life changes so does your body's requirements, so when you find this expert, create an amazing relationship with him or her, as he will be your family's best friend for many years to come!

Because we live in a world where there is a drug for every symptom and we are severely over medicated, I want to be very clear that whole-food supplements are NOT like drugs nor do they act like drugs. In fact, you can find yourself taking six (tablets, capsules, pills, etc.) of any one supplement because these supplements are entirely food based and there are no fillers or additives. And if you find yourself taking multiple supplements, then you're going to find yourself taking a handful of supplements in the morning and in the evening. I bring this to your attention because the majority of people relate taking pills to taking medications, and of course, you're not supposed to take handfuls of medications or you may overdose. There is no such thing as overdosing on whole-food supplements. It would be like eating too much! Having said that, I don't encourage that you purposely take more than the recommended dosage as you'll just be wasting your money and causing your body to work overtime to excrete the extra nutrients that your body can't use at that very moment.

3. Fitness

> "Fitness is like a relationship. You can't
> cheat and expect it to work."
> **Ultra Healthy Mindset**

Fitness plays a vital role in overall health. To be clear and to reiterate, there is a huge difference between being fit (looking good and feeling good) and being healthy. There are people out there who are extremely fit (they workout daily, eat clean, and avoid the habits of a poor lifestyle), and yet they're suffering from chronic diseases and symptoms that are minimizing their quality of life. There are fit people all over the world suffering from chronic and fatal diseases. You can look great on the outside and even feel good on the inside and still not be healthy. Being a marathon runner, I was a good example of this all the way up until my twenties. I looked lean, cut, and strong, yet on the inside, I was miserable, suffering, and my health was progressively worsening.

In fact, just recently I read about a local ultra-marathoner who died of a heart attack at the age of 37. Does that even make sense? Someone who is capable of running over 50 miles in a weekend losing his life to a heart attack is hard to comprehend. But if you understand that there is a vast difference between being fit and being healthy, that tragedy starts to make sense. When you understand how the body works, it makes complete sense how something like this can take place.

The big take away here is not to base your health on how you look and feel. If you're going to brush aside Function and only focus on Food, Fitness, and Fun you will look great while having fun short-term, but you will not be happy in the long run.

Fitness can be confusing and even a little scary. I want to be clear that I am not a certified fitness trainer nor am I proposing the one-size-fits-all workout. Ultimately you have to do what's right for you. The number one reason why people don't workout is because they never get started in the first place. They simply don't know what to do or where to start. They don't dare go to the gym in fear that they are going to stick out like a sore thumb. Nobody likes being the new person in any situation, let alone a gym where you're surrounded by fit people walking around in tight clothing, grunting, and throwing weights around. For this reason, I suggest you take baby steps just like you're going to do with food.

Here are the top three strategies that will be the foundation for moving your fitness level towards your health goals and ultimately experiencing extraordinary health:

3.1) Fitness Schedule – have dedicated time during the week to workout

3.2) Fitness Goals – use your goals to keep you motivated

3.3) Fitness Progression – include a form of accountability that measures your progression

Before we dive into the three fitness strategies that you will use to develop your roadmap, I want to revisit the story about the ultra-marathoner who suffered a heart attack. I believe that if you can fully comprehend this particular instance, you will be more aware of your body as you go through the many changes during your journey beyond symptoms.

So how exactly does a 37-year-old, extremely-fit male suffer and die from a heart attack in the first place? If the nerves that are sending strength and energy to the heart and lungs are compromised and irritated, those organs are not functioning to the best of their ability and are working overtime. If the heart is naturally working overtime and an athlete pushes his body beyond limits, then the heart is overexerted to the point where it's literally breaking down. If this 37-year-old was an athlete his entire life all the way back into his childhood, then there is a strong chance that for the past 25-30 years, his heart had been working harder than it needed to and was aging quicker than he physically was. So by the time a seven-year-old boy ages 30 years, his heart may have aged up to 60 years, and now you have a 37-year-old ultra-marathoner beating up a heart that is functioning at a level of a 67-year-old. By working out and doing what he felt was great for his health, he was ultimately breaking his body down and literally killing himself. The moral of this story is that if you're going to be physically active (which I highly encourage you to do) and beat your body up, you need to take care of your body and ensure that it's functioning at its peak performance. This is especially true for children who are active in sports, gymnastics, dance, etc.

There are endless celebrities who you can relate this to as well. Go ahead and Google Patrick Swayze and Farah Fawcett for starters. I don't think anyone would argue that these two stars looked good in their prime. As you look through their photos you will see that they were fit and beautiful looking. As movie stars, they made a ton of money and were able to afford the healthy lifestyle. They could afford to invest in personal trainers, nutrition experts, coaches, and have the best of the best doctors take care of them. Now, what happened to both of these actors? They ended up developing, suffering from, and ultimately dying from cancer. We're all aware that cancer does not occur overnight. This is the importance of creating then achieving your 30-year goals. I assure you neither of these two Hollywood actors intended to die of cancer at such a young age. This is why not basing your health on how you look and how you feel is so important.

Fitness is the third Foundational Principle of Health. Fitness plays a vital role in your overall health but takes a back seat to Function and Food.

3.1 Fitness Schedule

"The key is not to prioritize what's on your schedule,
but to schedule your priorities."
Stephen Covey

Start small and dedicate the appropriate time during the week so that workouts are a priority. Ultimately, you want to develop a routine where fitness will become a regular part of your day. That time must be set in stone and nothing can interfere with it, so plan accordingly. Once you have a time set aside, you need to have the resources to be able to work out. Will you be running outside, riding a bike, lifting at a gym, joining a class, following along to a workout video at your home, etc.? Whatever you choose is fine. Stick with your workout for a minimum of one month, and at the end of that month, you will know whether you enjoy that workout or if you need to find something else. No matter what you choose to do, the first two to three weeks will be the toughest. Stick with the plan and just do it, and you will begin to see results that will motivate you to keep going. You must force yourself to follow through for the first two to three weeks no matter what.

3.2 Fitness Goals

"Fitness is not about being better than someone else…
it's about being better than you used to be."
Ultra Healthy Mindset

The purpose of fitness is to provide you with strength, mobility, flexibility, and cardiovascular stability. Ultimately, fitness isn't about what you choose to do, as long as you're doing something. All forms of exercise work as long as you're willing to put in the work. You have to enjoy whatever form of physical exercise you choose, otherwise there is absolutely no way that you will stick with your fitness routine.

Your fitness routine will be determined primarily by your fitness goals. If you're an elite athlete competing at a professional level, then your workouts are going to have to be super intense and specific. If you're someone looking to put on some major muscle mass and be able to lift an extremely heavy weight, then you're going to have to bulk up by incorporating a specific lifting program to meet your goals. For the general public, working out three to four days a week will do the trick. And I'm not going to encourage a lengthy duration time for working out because, truthfully, it's possible for someone to get a better workout in 20 minutes than some will get in 75 minutes. Find out what works best for you, your goals, and your current schedule.

Your fitness goals can be treated much like your health goals. Think big, write them down, and view them often. Remember, if you're willing to work, your exercise program will work!

"My definition of fitness is to be able to carry out all of the activities in life that you desire plus have a physical reserve at the end of the day to do something besides lie down and flip the remote. If you can do all that, if you're functional, then you're fit. It doesn't matter if you have great abs or can bench-press your body weight. Those things have nothing to do with real life."
James Glinn, physical therapist, in an interview with Joe Kita for his 1999 book Wisdom of Our Fathers

3.3 Fitness Progression

"When you feel like quitting think about why you started in the first place."
Ultra Healthy Mindset

Once you get into a routine and are consistently working out, you can then begin to adjust your workouts and take them to the next level. There is always a next level!

The key to fitness progression is writing down all of your workouts. This also serves as accountability. Get yourself a fitness calendar where you jot down all of your workouts for each day. At any given time, you will be able to see an entire month's worth of workouts, and I promise you, seeing this calendar will make you feel amazing when you see the majority of the calendar filled with workouts. On the flip side, if you see too many empty days, the blanks spaces are going to serve as the accountability you need to get back on track.

Track every single detail so that you can compile all the data and be able to monitor your progression. Examples of what to write down include: your workout, how many reps you performed, how much weight you used, how long you did a particular exercise, the distance you were able to complete, etc. As you cycle through your workouts and begin to repeat them, you will be able to compare where you were and where you are. You need to be able to see that you are going up in weights or that you're running longer distances in shorter time periods. You will use this information much like you will use your goals: to motivate yourself to always want to improve yourself.

I personally workout six to seven days a week at the exact same time every day because it is a daily ritual that I have developed. My workouts tend to change throughout the year depending on what my goals are. When I'm training for a marathon, I focus on long-distance running as well as track workouts, and my weight can drop as low as 165lbs. When I'm in the mode of lifting heavy and putting on muscle mass, my weight can jump as high as 205lbs. When I'm not looking to compete in any races or events, I typically weigh180 lbs., and I'm doing very simple, non -intensive workouts in my home so that I can stay fit and maximize my health. Again, there is no right or wrong way to do this unless you have specific goals you are aiming for. For general health, I recommend you get into a routine that you enjoy so that you can maintain your strength, mobility, flexibility, and cardiovascular benefits.

4. Fun

"There's lots of people in this world who spend so much time watching their health that they haven't the time to enjoy it."
Josh Billings

The purpose of life is to experience happiness. Contrary to what most believe, the opposite of happy is not unhappy or sadness, rather it's boredom. If you find yourself regularly bored in life, you're clearly not as happy as you could be. Happiness is a choice. You can choose to be happy or you can choose to be miserable. The easiest way to be happy is to enjoy what you do and have fun doing it. Because you get to choose what you do in life, ultimately you get to choose whether you're happy or not. The more you are able to strengthen your mindset, the easier applying this "happiness" principle to your life will be.

If you're not having fun on a regular basis, you need to start rethinking what you do day to day throughout the week. If that requires you get a new job, then I strongly encourage you to rethink your career. If you're in a dysfunctional relationship, then consider breaking ties and finding someone who treats you the way you deserve to be treated. Remember, stress attacks the weakest part of your body, so if you're not happy and having fun, you're more than likely stressed out. Because you are making health a top priority and you have committed to do anything and everything to be healthy, give yourself permission to go find something or someone who brings you joy on a daily basis.

The key to having fun, experiencing joy, and being successful at all areas of life is relationships. This key is why your environment is so important. If you build strong, trusting relationships with people who love you, support you, and hold you accountable, you are going to do things in life that you never dreamed possible. Your environment is going to play a huge role in the success you have during your journey beyond symptoms.

The most important relationship in your life is the relationship you have with your significant other. Now I am not a relationship expert, however I will admit that my wife and I have put countless hours and have invested thousands and thousands of dollars into our relationship. The time and energy we have put into each other has dramatically increased our success and happiness in life. There is no greater support system than being on the same page and sharing a vision with your other half. If you are supported by your life-partner and have upfront agreements with one another, you will be unstoppable and there won't be a goal you cannot achieve, including your 30-year health goals. If you feel like you could use some suggestions for strengthening your love relationship, please read chapter fifteen.

What about having fun with your health goals? I'd like to outline the three ways I think there are to have more fun with your health goals.

First, be around and associate with like-minded people. Personally, I don't think you'll find a better place than a chiropractic office. The people in a Corrective Care Chiropractor office are all there because they want to be there, and they want to function to the best of their ability. Why would you not want to be a part of that type of energy?

Second, partner up with a friend. Friends make everything better, and you'll have a ton of fun with a friend when you begin getting creative with healthy food options, experimenting with meals and smoothies that you've never tried before. In addition, your friend will keep you motivated and on track to hit your health goals.

What's more fun than one friend? More friends! There are endless activities that you can do in a group setting. For example, you can play volleyball, soccer, softball, or any other organized sport. You can swim, rollerblade, run, or play on obstacle courses.

Third, make your health goals a game and compete with your partner or with yourself. If you're playing in a sports league or competing with a friend, the thrill of the competition may be fun for you. On the other hand, if you're not big into competition with others, you can play a game or compete with yourself to add more fun into your food prep or exercise routine. For example, how fast can you prepare your meals for the day? Make a game out of your meal prep and see if you can beat your time from yesterday. The same holds true for the number of reps you do in a given set or the amount of time you take to complete a run. Make things fun by turning your goals into a game.

There are more ways to have fun with your health goals, but these three are a start. Personally, when I work out alone, I have fun listening to music and podcasts. My workouts leave me feeling happy and accomplished which leads to a great day. Remember, the happier you are, the less stressed out you are.

Application Exercise #6

Now that you are aware of the Core Four Principles, grade yourself on each individual category using a scale from one to ten. Determine where you score the lowest and where you may need to focus as we begin to build the strategy portion of your Roadmap to Extraordinary Health. This is an extremely important exercise that will build the foundation for you to reach your three-month health goals. (You can download "The Core Four Foundational Principles of Health" scale at InspiredToBe-Healthy.com)

Function

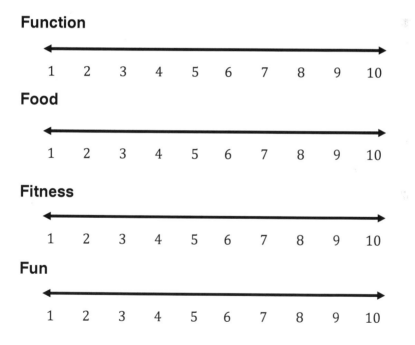

Food

1 2 3 4 5 6 7 8 9 10

Fitness

1 2 3 4 5 6 7 8 9 10

Fun

1 2 3 4 5 6 7 8 9 10

Mentoring Moment

Game Changer: The Core Four Foundational Principles of Health consists of Function, Food, Fitness, and Fun. These four principles essentially make up your lifestyle. If you want to be healthy and achieve your 30-year health goals, then you need to have the appropriate lifestyle in place that will lead you towards those goals.

If you can give yourself an honest assessment of where you've been, where you currently are, and where you would like to be in each of the four individual categories of the Core Four, you will be able to put the strategy in place to be able to move forward in the six-step cycle of the Roadmap to Extraordinary Health! The key is to focus on the entire Core Four because experiencing extraordinary health if even one of the four is lacking is impossible.

Own It: After completing the Application Exercise, take the principles that you learned and teach them to someone else. If you can teach them, you will own them. If you own them, you're absolutely going to apply them to your life. Take the time to understand all of the Core Four, and introduce those concepts to the people closest to you in your life so that they too can begin to put a strategy in place that will allow for them to shift their lifestyles into a more proactive direction.

11
Step 4: Accountability
Build a Healthy
Environment

"You are the average of the five people
you spend the most time with."
Jim Rohn

I f you've made up your mind that you would like to be full of life and live a super healthy lifestyle, I will warn you that you need to start being very selective about where you get your health advice. If you tell someone that you are reading a book about how to become super healthy and experience extraordinary health, that person will most likely smile at you and then go into details of why getting super healthy is next to impossible to do - especially for you.

Give it a try! Meet up with a few friends, and I assure you at least one of them will make excuses for you of why YOU aren't able to be healthy and why YOU will never make the necessary lifestyle changes.

Part of the problem is that most people get health advice from family or friends who are struggling with or who have given up on being healthy. Most of the advice we get about health is from people close to us who either have been diagnosed with a disease themselves or who have a poor, unhealthy lifestyle. Some of the people you get advice from have never even thought being healthy was possible, let alone living a super healthy lifestyle.

You must look beyond the negative advice of friends, television, social media, blog's, "Get Healthy Quick" programs, and all the nonsense of there's-a-pill-for-every-symptom commercials and magazine articles.

Look beyond all the noise and confusion about health, and you will discover a select group of people who have created super healthy lifestyles and are experiencing an extraordinary quality of life. Like magnets of health, fitness, and happiness, these people appear to magically have more energy, more vitality, and be more productive no matter what happens. They somehow manage to thrive in the "bad times." These are the people you should study and model your health habits on.

I tell you this because early on in my life, my environment influenced me, and I adopted the philosophies of those closest to me. I grew up eating fast food, cereal, snacks, candy, pop, and essentially all the foods I shouldn't have been eating. On top of that, my dad was a smoker. Both my mother and father were both brought up without the realization of what health really was. By no fault of their own, our family quickly fell into the reactive system of healthcare that led to the vicious cycle of chasing symptoms and ultimately depending on the regular use of medications.

Typically, parents raise their kids the same way they were raised. Looking down the line, your great-great-grandpa raised your great-grandpa the way that he was raised. Your great-grandpa raised your grandpa the way that he was raised. And the same goes for grandpa raising your dad, and ultimately, your dad raising you. For those of you who have children, you most likely are raising your child either how you or your spouse were raised. You simply don't know what you don't know.

You must be willing to destroy everything in your life that is not excellent. Don't let anyone tell you health is not possible. Family, friends, acquaintances, leaders... don't let them tell you that what you're trying to do for you and your family is not possible. You don't want to be that person thirty years down the road who is bitter, miserable, or angry at the world, wishing you would have done something differently.

Health is often an emotional topic of conversation. We all know people close to us who have suffered or are currently suffering from a health condition in which they were told there is nothing more they can do. Maybe that someone is you. The reality is that every single person in this world has his or her own crisis to deal with in life. I assure you, whatever that crisis may be that you have gone through or are currently going through, there is someone who has overcome a situation similar and even worse than yours in life. When the people close to you try to give you excuses for why you can't do something, find those people who have already achieved what you want to achieve. I promise that these people exist and there are a ton of them just waiting to help others who are seeking to do what they have done.

The top factors determining health are Lifestyle and Environment. Beginning to achieve your 12-month goals will lead you to take charge of your Lifestyle, and the goal of this chapter is to focus on creating a healthy Environment that will support you during your journey.

Growth happens naturally in the right atmosphere. That's why you must surround yourself with the people and resources that will help you get there. There is too much negativity in the world we live in, and you will constantly be bombarded by all the negativity if you don't plan and create your own positive, supportive environment.

So, let's start by limiting the stress in your life and creating a non-stressful and supportive environment that will help you thrive and push you to grow into the person you aim to be.

"It always seems impossible until it's done."
Nelson Mendella

The Makeup of Your Healthy Environment

Why You Need a Healthy Environment?

"If you have health, you probably will be happy, and if you have health and happiness, you have all the wealth you need, even if it is not all you want."
Elbert Hubbard

The American lifestyle is "go, go, go, now, now, now" – how much can I get done today? We've created this vicious, stressful cycle we call "everyday life," and it's literally killing us. We need to be able to create a non-stressful environment to help us slow down and keep our minds from being distracted by nonproductive and even harmful thoughts.

If you're routinely in a healthy, supportive environment, you will be setup for success, and staying focused, being productive, and succeeding will be that much easier.

I believe that the greatest definition of success is happiness. Success is not being skinny. Success is not having six-pack abs. Success is not having the ability to run a marathon. Success isn't even being able accomplish your health goals. Success is happiness. Success is enjoying life with the people you love. It's spending time with your kids or grandchildren. It's feeling fulfilled and serving your life purpose while helping others.

Put yourself in the right atmosphere, surrounded by the right people, and you will be happier, healthier, and more effective in life.

Who Is in Your Healthy Environment?

> "A bad cold wouldn't be so annoying if
> it weren't for the advice of our friends."
> ### Kin Hubbard

Who you hang out with is a big deal. Do you hang out with people who go to the gym or people who hang out at fast food joints? Do you hang out with people who get up early in the mornings to work out or people who are closing down the local bar night after night?

Do you hang out with positive people or negative people? If you choose to hang out with negative people who see the worst in everything and consistently tell you that you can't do what you want to do, you'll eventually believe what they're telling you, begin to buy into their B.S., and never achieve what you set out to do.

So, you must be careful and free yourself from negative people. They don't want you moving forward because if you're moving forward that means that they're moving backward. And they don't like that! The people who continuously try to pull you back are not your true friends. Your true friends will love you, encourage you, support you, and try to build you up. The more positive people you hang out with, the more you will believe in yourself... and the easier reaching your goals and becoming the person you wish to be will be.

If you hang out with cynical, negative, unhealthy people, you will end up negative and unhealthy. Always strive to get on top in life because it's the bottom that is overcrowded. You don't want to be on the bottom. Being on the bottom is easy, and being unhealthy doesn't take any effort. Staying unhealthy doesn't take any motivation or any drive.

Bottom line: you're going to have to make some uncomfortable decisions. If your friends or family members are negative ninnies, you need to consciously decide to limit your time with them. You may even have to drop a friend or two with the intentions that he or she is holding you back, and you simply can't grow with his dead weight clinging onto you. You deserve better.

And this kind of selectiveness doesn't stop with people closest to you. For example, if you routinely go to a medical doctor who seeks to find something wrong with you and recommends that you to take medications on a regular basis, then don't be surprised the next time you're there and you find yourself leaving with more prescriptions. Seek a health professional who is going to support your goals and push you to take responsibility for your health. If you regularly have appointments with professionals who seek to "save you" and give you excuses for all of your problems, offering you easy ways out (short-term gratification), then don't be surprised when that short-term gratification turns into long-term pain.

Surround yourself with people who support your 30-year vision. Surround yourself with people who are healthy or people who are at least on their way to being healthy. Surround yourself with people who you want to be like. Who is the fittest person you know? Who eats the healthiest? Who has the most fun? Those are the people you need to seek out and make regular fixtures in your life. The people who you surround yourself with are the people who you will become.

Lastly, your spouse plays a key role in your environment. He or she must share (or at least be open to the idea of sharing) your vision, especially if you see him as part of your vision. He must be healthy too. If your spouse is not on board, your roadmap is going to become confusing and almost unrecognizable as you face endless uncertainty. You may even experience numerous detours and several roadblocks during your journey.

What Is a Healthy Environment?

"The environment is everything that isn't me."
Albert Einstein

Focus on the objective... your long-term health is far more important than short-term gratification. Don't give in to the simple pleasures now if they don't contribute to your long-term objective. Ask yourself often, "Is what I'm about to do right now following my core values and contributing to my life vision?" Far too often, we fall victim to short-term gratification which leads to the demise of our long-term goals. The "What" portion of your Environment is your everyday surroundings that affect you on a daily basis.

You now know what health is and how the body works. If you have a medicine cabinet in your home, that's a problem. You now know that stress attacks the weakest part of the body. Medications are a chemical stress to your body. Chasing symptoms simply doesn't work. Trying to convince yourself that you're not going to use the drugs that you pile in your medicine cabinet doesn't work; the reality is that if you buy medications and they're in your home, you're going to use them. Ditch the medicine cabinet and all the drugs inside of it, and create a Health Cabinet filled with supplements, homeopathy, essential oils, herbs, etc.

The same goes with the food and beverage products in your home. If you buy and fill your refrigerator, freezer, cabinets, and pantry full of junk food and treats, all that junk food will get eaten. If you buy massive amounts of alcohol, soda pop, ice cream, snacks, candy, etc., you're going to consume them. Another reason why meal planning and food prep, discussed in chapter nine, are so important.

You need to take the time to break down the products that you use on a daily basis as this plays a vital role in your environment. If you surround yourself with temptations that you know are not good for you long-term, developing good rhythms and rituals that will contribute to a healthy lifestyle are going to be extremely difficult for you.

Some examples of the products that you use and surround yourself with every day that you will want to look into and purchase quality items include: food products, supplements, cleaning products, personal care items, water, dishes, food storage containers, cookware, etc.

Are you taking the generic supplements from your local retail store because you came across a two for one deal? Or are you taking the higher-quality, whole-food supplements that will provide you with the best chance to function, heal, and get stronger?

Are you purchasing the standard cleaning products that are chemically toxic because you simply don't know the difference and that's what everyone else buys? Or are you going the natural route and spending a few extra bucks on products that are going to clean just as good and not expose you or your family to the chemical stresses that over time will breakdown your body and ultimately affect your health?

Are you using the everyday, standard, personal-care items and exposing yourself to massive chemical toxins? Your skin is your largest organ, and paying attention to what you're putting on your skin (as these products will absorb into your body) is imperative. The rule is if you won't put it in your mouth, you shouldn't put it on your skin. The big items to watch for are makeup, lotions, soaps, shampoo and conditioner, toothpaste-fluoride, hair products, deodorant, and certainly the water that is used in your household. I mentioned this earlier... one of the best investments you can make for you and your family's health is to get an entire home water filtration system so that you are drinking and showering with water that is pure and not full of toxic metals.

Are you storing your foods in toxic plastic containers or are you investing in safer glass containers? Are you cooking with pans that are coated with polytetrafluoroetheylen (PTFE) which turns into toxic Perfluorooctanoic acid (PFOA) at high heat, making these pans dangerous both for the cook and those eating the food? Or are you using cast iron or ceramic based pans that don't produce the toxins? Certain kinds of kitchenware have been proven to discharge toxic fumes and chemicals into your food. Over time these foreign substances can build up in your body and potentially damage your health.

In addition to the products that you use and surround yourself with every day, pay attention to the rest of your physical environment. The last thing you want to do is put yourself in an overwhelming, unorganized, stressful environment. Your home, car, office should be organized and give you a sense of pride, not overwhelm. The things you own should bring you joy and happiness. If they don't, get rid of them. The last thing you want is clutter. Declutter the areas that you spend the majority of your life in. Get rid of old clothes that you don't wear and anything else you keep just for the sake of keeping but really brings you no joy. There are multiple great resources out there that will walk you step-by-step on how to declutter your home so that you can get rid of the unneeded stress and focus on what brings you joy and fuels you to be better and more productive.

> "To find peace, sometimes you have to be willing
> to lose your connection with the people, places, and
> things that create all the noise in your life."
> **Ultra Healthy Mindset**

Where Can You Find or Create a Healthy Environment?

> "I think you might dispense with half your doctors
> if you would only consult Dr. Sun more."
> **Henry Ward Beecher**

The "Where" portion of your environment are the places you regularly visit. The places you visit play a massive role in your ability to accomplish and achieve your health goals.

The stressful environment of a hospital filled with sick people, where doctors and staff are performing reactive care, is certainly not a positive, thriving environment that will support your goals. A much better environment would be the office of a proactive, healthcare professional, where the doctors take time to teach and genuinely care for their patients. That is an environment that will have a much more of a positive effect on you reaching your health goals.

If you're in the habit of getting your morning coffee and checking your email at the local fast food joint, you will continue to eat processed, unhealthy foods and put poor fuel into your body. As opposed to having a good, strong morning routine that puts high quality fuel into your body and allows for you to be productive without any negative distractions.

Will your home offer what you need to be able to reach your fitness goals? Or do you need to incorporate a gym or fitness facility so that you have the environment that supports your fitness goals?

Do you do your grocery shopping at the local, discounted grocery store because buying canned and prepackaged foods is cheaper, or have you made the choice to shop at a Whole Foods store and invest in organic, non-GMO, fresh and raw foods that are of higher quality? An added benefit to shopping at Whole Foods is the people at Whole Foods tend to be the people who have similar health tendencies as you're striving for, whereas those shopping at the local discount grocery store tend to be the people with a mindset that is not focused on health as a top priority.

Are you going to a Corrective Care Chiropractic office because you know that is where you will have the best chance to function to the best of your ability? Or are you going to the chiropractor down the road who gives the exact same treatment to every single patient that walks into his or her office regardless of why that patient is there because the office accepts your insurance? My recommendation is that you go to the doctor that tells you what you need to hear and not necessarily what you would like to hear.

Application Exercise #7

Don't do what most people do and try to "make do" with your current environment. Do not limit yourself. You were born to be healthy. You were born to be excellent. You were born to make a difference. Surround yourself with people who see greatness in you and integrate into an environment where you can thrive.

To help you with this, answer the following questions: (You can download the "Building a Healthy Environment" worksheet at InspiredToBeHealthy.com)

Does the environment at your home support you being the best you?

Do your relationships support you becoming the best you?

Does your place of work inspire you to be better?

Do your extra-curricular activities allow you to have fun and grow as a person?

Do the people who are closest to you (the people you interact with every single day) support a healthy positive growing environment?

Does your home allow you to be healthy and focus on what's important to you, or are you surrounded by clutter, television, and technology that distract you as well as junk food that gives you urges and cravings?

Are you constantly receiving push back? What is routinely stressing you out?

Who is criticizing you for wanting to be better? Who is constantly seeing the negative in everything you do? These are the people, places, and things that you need to be willing to separate yourself from. I am not asking that you quit them cold turkey. Instead, I am asking you be real with yourself, so you can begin to separate yourself from the people, places, and things that are holding you back from being the person you were destined to be.

Truthfully, as you begin to strengthen your mindset and create positive habits, these people, places, and things will naturally begin to fade away from you in the sense that they're going to be uncomfortable seeing you become better.

In the beginning, though, identifying these negative attributes in your environment is important. So, take a moment now and make an inventory list of where you spend most of your time and with whom. Do these people and places encourage, support, and motivate you towards your health goals? If not, then perhaps you need to make some adjustments. Which people and places do you need to begin limiting your time or possibly remove from your life all together?

1. _____   4. _____

2. _____   5. _____

3. _____   6. _____

Now, make a list of people and places you think you should be hanging out with and at? Where do you need to start going and who do you need to start spending more quality time with?

1. _____   4. _____

2. _____   5. _____

3. _____   6. _____

You must make creating your healthy environment a top priority, an environment that acknowledges you for what you do and that appreciates you for who you are. Create an environment for yourself where you can continuously progress and feel encouraged to achieve your 30-year health goals.

Mentoring Moment

Game Changer: Your Environment serves as your accountability to your health goals. Surrounding yourself with the right people, resources, and atmosphere that will support you and encourage you to reach your health goals is vital. If you are to complete the journey beyond symptoms, achieve your 30-year health goals, and experience extraordinary health, your environment must be top notch.

Surround yourself with people who you would like to be like. Surround yourself with the resources that will allow you to better yourself and give you an honest chance of reaching your goals. Lastly, live in an atmosphere that excites you and drives you to be better. Growth is the purpose of this journey. If you are to accomplish what you set out to accomplish, your 30-year vision, you simply can't accomplish your health goals on your own, so take this step seriously and make moving forward easier on yourself!

Own It: To get the most out of this chapter, complete the Application Exercise so you understand how your current environment has been affecting you and how the new environment you're going to begin to build for yourself will help you reach your health goals. Take the principles that you learned and teach them to someone else. If you can teach them, you will know them. If you know them, you're absolutely going to apply them to your life.

12
Step 5: Take Action
Develop Self-Discipline

"The path to success is to take massive, determined action."
Tony Robbins

You know your goals, and you know what you must do to reach those goals. Now it's time to take action and stay on track by developing self-discipline.

Discipline equals freedom. The more discipline you have the more freedom you have. To most people, this sounds counterintuitive. Most people think if you are living a disciplined lifestyle that you have no freedom. In reality, having self-discipline gives you more time and freedom because you have the discipline to get up earlier in the morning. You'll have more money because you have financial discipline to save and live below your means. You'll have more success because you have the discipline to accomplish your tasks and goals.

Does having discipline mean that you'll be perfect and never slip up? No. We're human. Making mistakes and slipping up are a part of life. But having self-discipline will help you stay on track more often than not.

So, how do you develop self-discipline? Developing self-discipline starts with how you view yourself. Are you the type of person who sets a goal and achieves it? Are you the type of person who will do whatever it takes to reach your goals? Are you the type of person who will do the uncomfortable activities needed to achieve your goals?

Notice that I didn't say, "Have you been the type of person to... ." I said, "Are you the type of person to... ."

Look, since reading this book, you're starting to become a different person. You don't have to be the type of person you used to be. You can now be the person you want to be: the type of person you know you deserve to be and the type of person you know you must be in order to achieve your 30-year goals.

So, who are you and who do you have to be to reach your 30-year goals? Let's explore the answers to this question...

Application Exercise #8

To help you express who you are – the type of person who can and will achieve any goal in life – write down ten reasons why you will not fail at achieving your 30-year health goals. Here are some examples to help you get started:

"I will absolutely achieve my health goals because..."

...I am disciplined. I am determined. I am committed.

...I am making myself a priority.

...I don't know how to fail. And even if I did, I wouldn't be any good at it!

...I said I would and my word is my honor.

...my WHY is far greater than any force, excuse, or reason I could come up with.

...I have a supportive environment that will encourage me and hold me accountable.

...there are too many people counting on me and I don't dare let them down.

Your turn. Write down ten reasons why you will not fail at achieving your 30-year health goals:

"I will absolutely achieve my health goals because..." (You can download the "Building Your Affirmations" worksheet at InspiredToBeHealthy.com)

1. _____   6. _____

2. _____   7. _____

3. _____   8. _____

4. _____   9. _____

5. _____   10. _____

Congruent, Consistent Action

"The distance between your dreams
and reality is called action."
Ultra Healthy Mindset

Like I mentioned above, developing self-discipline starts with how you view yourself. The next step to develop self-discipline is to realize this fact: the actions you take must be congruent and consistent with who you are and what you're trying to accomplish.

So, when your alarm goes off in the morning, get up. Don't lie in bed wondering if you should get up. Get up! Making this decision will impact you for the rest of the day and help you flex your decision-making muscle first thing in the morning.

Nobody wants to get up in the morning, but ultra-healthy people do. The ultra-healthy would love to hit the snooze button and crawl back into their warm, cozy bed. But they don't. Why? Because ultra-healthy people get up and live each day on purpose, and they have developed self-discipline that's congruent with who they are and the goals they're trying to achieve.

When you have the decision to watch TV or take the time to work on your body, choose to take care of your body and exercise. When you have the decision to hit the drive-thru and grab a quick meal or make yourself a healthy, nutritious meal, choose the healthy meal. When you're under the weather and you have the decision to focus on your symptoms or clearing your body of subluxations so your body can heal itself, choose optimal function over drugs.

You'll be faced with these types of decisions every day. How you move forward with each decision will determine your lifestyle and ultimately your health. It's just like the old axiom, "Actions speak louder than words." Saying you want something is easy, but achieving what you want takes hard work and discipline. The decisions you make and the actions you take each and every day show you and your loved ones the person you are.

Understanding that life is not going to slow down or stop whether you make the right decision to reach your goals or not is important. Life doesn't slow down. Time moves forward whether we like it or not. The key is to keep consistent with and stay focused on our short and long-term goals, so you can be the person you know you are and achieve the goals you've set for yourself.

Make the decision and commitment to take congruent, consistent actions.

Setting Yourself Up for Success

"You are what you do, not what you say you'll do."
Ultra Healthy Mindset

Self-discipline will help you follow through with what you need to do to function to the best of your ability. Self-discipline will help you make consistent and better decisions about the food you eat. Self-discipline will help you work out regularly and achieve your fitness and health goals. And most importantly, self-discipline will allow you to live the life that you were designed to live, to help you reach your life vision, and have fun and be healthy while doing it!

However, just because you know self-discipline will help you achieve all of this and more doesn't mean you'll start your day tomorrow being more disciplined. That's why I want to help you set yourself up for success and give you a few strategies to start using discipline to your advantage and stay disciplined from here on out.

First, I suggest taking ten to fifteen minutes in the morning and getting emotionally engaged with your goals. A good way to do this is to do a visualization exercise. How? By spending some time visualizing your future as if you're already living it. What does your future-self look like? How does your future-self feel? Walk yourself through your ideal future and verbally describe everything you see, smell, taste, and feel. What and who do you see around you? What do you smell in your environment? What do you feel like in your surroundings? What do you hear in the background? Try this out right now. Then, use this simple yet powerful technique every morning to emotionally engage yourself with your goals.

You don't have to stop there, though. You can also use that time in the morning to read some affirmations out loud. Do you recall the Application Exercise we did earlier? Use my examples and the ones you created as your initial affirmations. For example, say to yourself...

"I will absolutely achieve my health goals because I am disciplined."

"I will absolutely achieve my health goals because I am making myself a priority."

"I will absolutely achieve my health goals because I don't know how to fail. And even if I did, I wouldn't be any good at failing!"

"I will absolutely achieve my health goals because I said I would and my word is my honor."

"I will absolutely achieve my health goals because my WHY is far greater than any force, excuse, or reason I could come up with."

"I will absolutely achieve my health goals because I have a supportive environment that will encourage me and hold me accountable."

Feel the words that you are saying. Believe the words that you are saying. Doing so will reinforce these positive thoughts and tell your brain what to focus on. Also, remind yourself why your 30-year health goals are so important to you and why your life-style is the stepping stone to get you there. Think about how great your future is going to be when you reach those goals and you're living your life vision. Let that vision sit in your heart and really feel the satisfaction and excitement of the journey, get enthusiastic about your vision. If your heart is disengaged, being disciplined will be difficult.

Another strategy you can use is to setup blocks of time through-out the day that you work on yourself. Those times are for you and should be used for only you. For example, your workout time would be one of these blocks of time. Another block of time could be when you prepare your meals or when you per-form your spinal hygiene. And yet another time could be when you put the kids to bed and focus on your significant other or reflect on your day (what went well and what needs more at-tention), so you go to bed not trying to juggle a million ideas.

One more strategy you can use is to end your day by writing out your schedule for the next day. That way, you can schedule yourself first before anyone or anything gets in your way. Re-member, this is your life and you must schedule the things that are important to you. Scheduling your day the night before will help you stay off social media, keep you away from email, and hold you back from turning on the TV the next morning. I can-not stress how important this schedule is. The minute you en-gage in something else you are no longer on your agenda and you are reacting to someone else's agenda. Getting your brain back on track to focus on you after you've lost that focus is very difficult.

Discipline Does Get Easier

Your decision to stay disciplined will get easier. Yes, the first two to three weeks starting your new program will be the hardest. But forcing yourself to follow your roadmap for three weeks no matter what is going on in your life and regardless of what you are feeling is imperative.

Why? Because after those first three weeks, you will begin to feel different. You will notice a change in yourself. This change will provide you with the motivation to proceed and continue to pursue your short-term goals. And this motivation will carry you and keep you wanting to continue to follow your roadmap.

Just like your biceps muscles grow with every set of biceps curls you perform, your discipline muscle grows with every decision you make. And the more useful decisions you make to achieve your goals, the easier staying on track and being disciplined will become.

Mentoring Moment

Game Changer: Find joy in discipline! Discipline helps you get things done. Discipline equals freedom. The more discipline you have, the more freedom you will have. Self-discipline is arguably the most powerful characteristic when it comes to personal growth and development. With self-discipline, your journey to extraordinary health will become enjoyable and you will feel accomplished while reaping the benefits of living the lifestyle that you have created for yourself!

If you have not done so already, take the time to complete the Application Exercise. Until you are naturally and easily living the lifestyle that you have developed, keeping your vision, your WHY, and your 30-Year Health Goals at the forefront of your mind is imperative. Your Top Ten Reasons will serve as fuel to keep you fired up and pushing towards what you know you're capable of.

Own It: To get the most out of this chapter, take the principles that you learned about discipline and teach them to someone else. If you can teach them, you will have a better understanding of what it takes to be self-disciplined and begin to develop and make this characteristic a part of who you are. This will have a tremendous impact on your life and certainly on your journey to extraordinary health.

13

Step 6: Celebrate & Refocus - Living Your Ideal Lifestyle

"A healthy lifestyle not only changes your body, it changes
your mind, your attitude and your mood."
Ultra Healthy Mindset

The best way to stay motivated and disciplined is to celebrate your victories along the way. Far too often we want
to reach our destination without experiencing the journey. But
that's not how life works. Life is a series of journeys. What you
experience along the way is what shapes who you are in life.
Enjoying the journey and appreciating every milestone along
the way to achieving your goals is important. But that's sometimes easier said than done. After all, since we keep ourselves
so busy with our crazy, fast-paced lifestyles, pressing on without noticing or celebrating our victories is far too easy. However, I feel that celebrating your victories is necessary and will
help you achieve your goals faster. Why? Because you'll set a
pattern in your mind of work-result-reward, and this pattern
will lead you to wanting and achieving more.

You see, that's where some people fall short. They never reward themselves for the good work they're doing and the goals they're achieving. Unfortunately, this tells their brains that their achievements are "no big deal," and their brains don't anchor work to results and results to rewards. A simplistic example of this is when you reward a child for a job well done. For example, if your children take out the trash, a simple, "great job!" or enthusiastic high-five (reward) will anchor or link the result you want to the work they did. Not saying anything to your children after they take out the trash won't create a link or anchor to the work, and thereby telling their brains that the work wasn't valued.

Application Exercise #9

We can use the same psychology to achieve our health goals by setting up a reward system. So, how do you set up a rewards system? It's simple. First, rewards are determined by what gets you excited. Do you like to read? You can reward yourself with an hour of alone time to read your favorite book once you achieve one of your small goals. Do you enjoy camping? You can reward yourself with a camping trip once you achieve a bigger goal. Again, your rewards should be based on what you enjoy. Take a moment now and write down a list of things you enjoy. Don't overcomplicate this. Jot down some ideas of what you can reward yourself with – big and small.

1. _____   5. _____

2. _____   6. _____

3. _____   7. _____

4. _____   8. _____

Next, take the goals you created earlier in this book and jot down a few milestones you can achieve on your way to achieving your goal. For example, if one of your goals is to go from 220 pounds down to 180 pounds in three months, you can have a milestone for every ten pounds you drop.

Finally, take your milestone goals and your rewards and link them together. So, when the scale hits 210 pounds, you can reward yourself with an hour to yourself to read. When you hit the 200-pound mark, you can reward yourself with a healthy dinner out on the town. When you hit the 190-pound mark, you can reward yourself with a "maid service" cleaning your house. And when you hit your three-month goal and drop to 180 pounds, you can reward yourself with an overnight trip to your favorite campgrounds.

As you can see, the first couple milestones get rewarded with small celebrations and the last couple get rewarded with bigger celebrations.

Take some time now to create your reward system. (You can download the "Creating Your Reward System" worksheet at InspiredToBeHealthy.com)

Refocus

I've helped thousands of clients over the years achieve their health goals (some you've read about in this book), and I'd be remiss if I didn't mention two eventualities that happen to every single person on their journey to extraordinary health...

1. You will have distractions.

2. You will have moments of complacency.

The key is to stay focused on your current goals until they are achieved, and then continue to reach for bigger and better goals. Life is a cycle. You'll set goals, get distracted, course-correct, and continue the process until you achieve your goals. Then, you'll start all over again.

So, you've already set your goals. Now, take action until you achieve them. Will you get side-tracked and distracted? Of course, you will. Keep your WHY in front of you and stay the course. By taking congruent, consistent action, you will eventually hit your goals.

Once you've achieved a goal, don't let complacency sink in. Start back at step one in this book and follow along to get your mindset right, reset your next batch of goals, and take action to achieve them. I assure you, by the time you end up back here at step six again, you will be a completely different person than you are now.

Rinse and repeat until you're the person you want to be, and you're living the healthy life you desire and deserve.

"Love yourself enough to live a healthy lifestyle."
Ultra Healthy Mindset

Mentoring Moment

Game Changer: Celebrating your small victories will change your life. You must acknowledge the things you have accomplished, appreciate yourself for who you're becoming, and celebrate your achievements. And when you set out for an even bigger goal, you must refocus your attention and energy so that you're setup for success for the next battle.

Own It: To get the most out of this chapter, take the principles that you learned and teach them to someone else. Better yet, share a goal you've recently accomplished with someone, and go out and celebrate together. Enjoy your accomplishment and reflect on how reaching your goal has changed the quality of your life already. Begin thinking about what the next level looks like and start drafting up your next set of goals. Once you have your new target, refocus and shoot away!

14
Transformational Rituals

"You will never change your life until you
change something you do daily. The secret
of your success is found in your daily routine."
John C. Maxwell

You now know the Six Steps to live an extraordinary life. Like I mentioned in the last chapter, all you have to do now is repeat the Six Steps until you're the person you want to be and you're living the healthy life you desire and deserve.

To help you speed up the process, here are four strategies that if you implemented them tomorrow and developed into regular habits, rhythms, and eventually daily rituals, they would allow you to regain your youth and vitality and take your life to an entirely new level:

1. Power Hour

2. Fitness Hour

3. Morning Ritual

4. Fidelity Hour

Power Hour – How to Create A Strong Mind and Be Spiritually Connected

Most people wake up and focus on the grueling stuff they had to go through yesterday, all the things that never got accomplished, and all the people they had to deal with. This is not how you want to start off your days. With all that you are trying to accomplish and achieve, you need to be better focused and your energy levels need to be up. This is the purpose of a Power Hour.

A Power Hour is the first hour after you awaken in the morning. This is the hour where you are encouraged to be selfish and devote this time to better understand who you are and where you're going. This is the hour you will develop yourself, sharpen your mind, and prepare your body for the day. And this is also the hour you will destress yourself for the day.

In other words, your Power Hour is meant to help you avoid the unintentional mornings of stress and chaos, so you can wake up each morning with a purpose and an intention. Your Power Hour will help you build you up, so you are strong and nothing will stand in your way.

The first twenty minutes of the day will determine the rest of your day, so starting the day off with gratitude is important. Every morning when your feet hit the floor, tell yourself that today is going to be a great day. Be thankful for the day that lies ahead of you and for all that you have in life. The easiest way to develop this habit is by placing your alarm clock far away from your bed so that you must get up to turn off the alarm. At that point, begin your gratitude and happy thoughts.

You want to break the habit of being grumpy, groggy, and cursing every beep of the alarm clock. You want to break the habit of hitting the snooze button and rolling back into bed. And you want to break the habit of checking your phone for social media, news, or email alerts. This hour is dedicated to you, not all the distractions of the world. Jumping out of bed and ignoring your phone is a temporary price to pay for the glory of a beautiful morning and, ultimately, an amazing day.

Your Power Hour should take place in an area of your home that is stress-free, relaxing, and has great energy. Take advantage of the complete silence and let your brain wonder. Create a to-do list that will allow you to be productive throughout the day and will make you feel accomplished at the end of the day. Write out your intentions for the day so that you have direction. And when you have your to-do list written out, don't focus on all of the tasks that need to get done, focus on who you have to be to ensure that list gets done. Visualize what you'd like to happen, and set yourself up to win. If you have direction and you know where you're going, no matter what distractions you come across during the day, you will keep laser focused and do what you know you need to do.

Now, if you have something important going on that day, give that event some Attention and create an Intention. What do you want to have happen? Think about your intention. Meditate on your intention. Journal about your intention. Do whatever you feel helps you manifest your intention.

Personally, I like meditation. Meditation is particularly powerful in the morning because it primes your nervous system for the day. Meditation helps stimulate the parasympathetic (rest and digest) nervous system and calms the sympathetic (fight or flight) nervous system, so that you can start your day from a place of peaceful clarity.

If affirmations work for you, starting your day off with these small but powerful positivity-boosting words can literally re-wire your brain and alter the trajectory of your entire day.

Meditation and affirmations help you tune your body and brain to the frequency of your dreams, so you can become a magnet for all the things you want out of life. You can use them in conjunction by making a list of a dozen or so "I AM" statements and meditating on them. Here are some affirmation examples you can use:

I AM Strong

I AM Smart

I AM Healthy

I AM Fit

I AM Disciplined

I AM Extraordinary

I AM Responsible

I AM Motivated

I AM Focused

I AM Powerful

I AM Successful

Not all these affirmations may be true right now, but you need to invite the things into your life as if they already are.

Doing what's right for you is important. Happiness is your responsibility. There is never-ending "good" in this world, and there is also never-ending "bad" in this world. It's up to you to focus on the good. Your Power Hour is the time devoted to you in your life to continue to strengthen your mindset. Stay away from social media and the news. There is plenty of time in the day where you can fry your brain with negative information. This hour is about you.

One of the hardest things to do is to challenge your limiting beliefs: challenging the negative thoughts in your head and talking back to your brain every time it tries to protect you by thinking logically and keeping you "safe" by not allowing you to take risks or face your fears. The constant messages that we are bombarded by every single day are constantly shaping our thoughts and making this process tougher. We are being conditioned to believe what's "normal." The constant drug commercials giving us false hope of quick fixes, the photo-shopped fitness models showing us what we're supposed to look like, the relationship magazines explaining how normal partners are having sex 4.3 times per week. We are constantly surrounded by unrealistic expectations and therefore never feel good enough.

I learned very quickly that if I could change my brain, I could change my life. Study after study shows that self-esteem plays a vital role in the level of success one experiences. People who are constantly negative about everything and see the worst in anything and everything are people with lower self-esteem. This does not make them bad people, they simply need to become aware of this negativity cycle and make changing their brains a priority.

Unfortunately, because these people are so negative about everything, and maybe this is you, they believe that the idea of trying to change the brain is stupid. They get defensive, as if the idea of changing their brain is a criticism. They feel like they are getting attacked. How do I know this? Because I had to change my brain. In fact, I'm still doing changing my brain. I continue to improve my perspective by seeing the best in people and focusing on positive thoughts rather than seeing the negative in everything. If you can see the best in yourself, seeing the best in others will come more naturally.

My Typical Power Hour

Because my Power Hour is a daily ritual, I often wake up a minute or two before my alarm clocks goes off. My internal alarm goes off at 3:56 a.m. The minute my eyes open, I begin my gratitude. "Thank You! Thank You!! Thank You!!!" I throw on an exaggerated smile on my face and I tell myself, "Today is going to be a (enter superlative) day!"

I then throw on my workout clothes that are laid out from the night before, and I mosey downstairs. The first thing I do is consume a tablespoon of apple cider vinegar (mixed with water) on an empty stomach. This serves as a smack-in-the-face wakeup as well as having numerous health benefits, including digestion support. In addition, depending on the time of year, I may consume liquid herbs as part of my supplementation regime.

Lastly, I grab water before heading into my Power Hour spot. I make it a point to consume a 32 oz. mason jar of water during my Power Hour. Drinking water in the morning has countless benefits, such as firing up your metabolism, flushing out toxins, fueling your brain and body, and hydrating you for the entire day. I personally like to buy bottles of organic lemon and lime juice to change up the taste of my water.

My Power Hour takes place in my home office or in another room in our home that my wife and I call our "experience room"

– a room in our home that is designed as our getaway room, used for relaxation and to experience great energy. Whether my Power Hour is in my office or my experience room, I take advantage of the complete silence, and I let my brain wonder. The first thing I do is write out my day so that I don't have to think about my schedule again, and I can prioritize the most important things.

After writing down my to-do list, my brain is completely free and I let it wonder. My most creative time is in the morning. I remind myself that "I AM the master of my thoughts! I determine how I feel!" I close my eyes, and I take three, deep breaths lasting nearly 90 seconds each. I put a big smile on my face for roughly a minute, and I take the time to feel the peace and gratitude in my heart and in the core of my body. Lastly, I start to program my brain for the success of the day, "Today I will absolutely get all the following tasks done," and I repeat the to-do list that I already created. I visualize myself accomplishing all my tasks with ease and enjoying every minute of my day. I know who I must be to ensure that it all gets done.

At that point, I am completely free and have 45 minutes to do whatever else I feel needs done. Often, I sit in silence, dreaming up ideas or just waiting until I'm told what it is I'm supposed to do. Other times, I choose to read. The main thing is I have no agenda, nor do I have any distractions. This is my time!

The habit of starting your day off with a positive attitude will grow you as a person and change your perspective on life. When you get your Power Hour down and it's a daily ritual that is clear and energizing, getting your mind right will get easier and easier until getting clear and calm will no longer take an hour but 30 seconds instead. When you've trained long enough and you're capable of changing your state at any given moment, life becomes easy. You stop taking things personally and when you're confronted with a challenge, you see the challenge for what it is instead of letting it interrupt your day. Everybody is confronted with challenges, and once you've conditioned your brain to view challenges as opportunities, you know there is something within you than can beat any challenge, overcome it, and then move forward as a result of it.

Fitness Hour – How to Get Physically Fit and Mentally Stable

You must keep your body moving. Don't wait until you're breaking down and unable to move with ease. Develop a routine that keeps you moving with ease. If I told you that I enjoy working out six to seven days a week, I would be lying to you. There are more days than not when I dread walking myself down into my gym, yet I do it because I know that working out is what my body needs.

There is no quick magic workout program that is going to allow you to hit your fitness goals and then never have to work out again in your life. Like with anything health related, it's about lifestyle. If you go and work out for the next 90 days straight, lose a bunch of weight, put on a ton of muscle mass, and look and feel better than you have in years - not having picked up any healthier habits along the way would be a bittersweet punchline. You can't bust your butt for a short period of time and expect to maintain those results if you go back to your old ways. If you would like to see change, you need to change what you've been doing.

The purpose of the Fitness Hour is to develop a rhythm that you can incorporate into your life that will allow you to get the movement your body needs on a regular basis without trying to make time during your already busy day to fit in a workout.

This is a rhythm that will hold you accountable and keep you physically fit no matter what stresses or curveballs life wants to throw at you. You can hit fitness goals and milestones that you never even thought possible if you will simply incorporate a Fitness Hour. Slow and steady is a heck of a lot better than throwing yourself into some big, bad, hardcore fitness program only to have yourself get overwhelmed, burnt out, or worse, injured.

Your personal Fitness Hour is something that you'll learn to cherish. Whether you complete a full, hour-long yoga session, a 30-minute run, or hit the weights, you will immediately feel the energizing, emotionally and mentally stimulating effect of moving your body in the morning.

I personally incorporate my workout immediately following my Power Hour in the mornings. Do I enjoy waking up at 3:56 a.m. every morning? Most days the answer is absolutely not. However, because health is a priority and I have developed my discipline muscle, I simply wake up that early because I know deep down that if I would like to serve my purpose in life to the best of my ability, I have to be the best me I can be. And that means getting my mind right and keeping my body fit. I promise you that developing these daily rituals is not hard. It may take some time and energy, but it's not hard and these rituals are beyond rewarding.

After my Power Hour, I refill my 32 oz. mason jar with water, I give five to ten minutes of my full, undivided attention to my wife before she heads out for her workout, and then I head down to my gym. My workouts are typically 45 minutes long, and I personally don't push my body past its limits. I document all of my workouts so that I can see the constant progression, and when I plateau after several weeks or even months, I like to change up my workouts.

Enjoying whichever type of workout you choose to incorporate is important. If you don't enjoy your workout, there's no chance you're going to stick with it. Choosing workouts that challenge you is also important.

I allot ten to twenty minutes after my workouts for Spinal Hygiene so that I can ensure that my body is functioning to the best of its ability. If you're going to physically beat your body up via workouts, taking care of your body and treating it with respect is extremely important. This is why I incorporate spinal hygiene immediately after my workouts; simply because there are no "ifs, ands, or buts" that my spinal hygiene will happen!

Lastly, when developing your Fitness Hour, it can be any time during the day that makes sense to you. I highly recommend that you choose a consistent time during the day when you will have no interruptions and no possibilities of something getting in the way from your taking that time for yourself. If there is a time that works for you every single day of the week, it will be easier for you to consistently do it without having to even think about it. On the flip side, it's not impossible, but less likely you're able to fit in your Power Hour if you have to change the time every day and try to fit it in where you have time. Your Power Hour should not be something you "try" to fit in during the day, it should be etched in and your day should be planned around it.

Morning Ritual – How to Get Grounded, Chemically Balanced, and Properly Fueled for the Day

To live a great life and to achieve your health goals, a morning ritual is absolutely vital. Studies show that people who start their mornings calm and happy finish the day in the same upbeat energized state. Whereas people who begin their days in a bad mood end their days feeling the same or worse. Furthermore, those who have elevated moods demonstrate higher productivity.

Build a routine that is right for you, that works for you, and that you can follow consistently. Don't leave any chance for thinking errors. Far too often, we get overwhelmed in the mornings. Give yourself ample time to get around. There's no surer way to ruin a day than to leave late and spend your morning rushing around.

If you build a morning ritual that works for you, you will accomplish more for yourself before your work day even begins than most do in an entire day. You will also set yourself up for success for the rest of the day!

There is no right or wrong when it comes to morning rituals, only what is right for you. So, I would like to show you my morning ritual so that you can start brainstorming and designing what's best for you.

After my Power Hour and my Fitness Hour, I head upstairs at 6:00 a.m. to get ready for the day. My window is short because whether I'm ready or not, I know that my kids will be waking up anywhere between 6:30-7:00 a.m., and they're usually ready for daddy's full attention. For this reason, I need to be on point and keep things moving!

One of the most important daily rituals that I have is listening to motivational audios while I brush my teeth, shave, shower, and floss. I simply use YouTube, and I listen to all of the self-empowering and motivational gurus. This strategy has been life -changing for me; it has literally changed my brain and my thought patterns. After so many years of listening to these type of audios, you begin to hear patterns and then quickly realize that they all say the same things, just from different perspectives. You then realize they're not telling you anything you don't already know; however, they're reminding you to be the best you can be, to push your fears aside, and let the real you come out. This is so important in a world where we are constantly bombarded with negativity, stress, and limitations. There is nothing more empowering than feeding your brain positivity on a daily basis. This positivity training is a must for anyone's morning ritual, so figure out where you can fit more positivity into your day.

Showering isn't only important for personal hygiene, but more importantly, it's a wakeup call for your mind and body, and taking a shower has been scientifically proven to stimulate creativity. If you want to take your showers to the next level, try taking cold showers. Although I don't love them, nor do I take them daily, a cold shower does have countless mental, physical, and emotional benefits.

Following a shower, another daily ritual that has endless benefits is the use of coconut oil. Use coconut oil as a lotion, focusing on your face, extremities, and guys can even use it in their hair. By the time I'm dried off, oiled up, and fully dressed, I'm typically greeted by my two, little, beautiful daughters, snuggling me and telling me how stylish I look.

The point is by the time I need to take care of the people in my life, I have over two-and-a-half hours that I have already poured into myself that I have used to better myself and allow me to continuously strive towards my 30-year health goals and my life vision!

Next, we head to the kitchen to load up on a plant-based breakfast. There's nothing better than a fresh, nutrient dense breakfast. I prefer a green smoothie with plant-based protein powder or eggs with leafy greens mixed in. There really are endless possibilities, you just need to be willing to get creative and stretch your boundaries of the typical breakfasts you currently have.

On top of a healthy nutritional breakfast, get in the ritual of taking your supplements with your breakfast. Make this a daily ritual and you won't ever have to worry about whether you remember to take them or not. You will naturally pull out your supplements and consume them because that's just what's done at breakfast time.

Your morning ritual is a wonderful time to meal prep for the day if you haven't already done so the night before. Set yourself up for success by building your veggie bowl for the day and packing a healthy lunch so that you have no excuses to impulse eat throughout the day. Aside from your veggie bowl and meals, be sure you have enough water packed to get you through the day. Remember, if you have it, you will consume it. If you don't intentionally pack water, and you take the nonchalant approach of drinking water when you're thirsty or when you "think of it," there's no way you will consume even close to enough water. Pack yourself 64 – 128 oz. of water for the day, and feel free to spruce your water up with organic lemon or lime juice to help yourself drink enough water.

If you are a coffee drinker, please note that 16 oz. of coffee is not the same as consuming 16 oz. of water. In fact, coffee has the opposite effect and dehydrates you. So, if you enjoy your coffee in the morning, just know that you will have to drink even more water throughout the day. If you have any bad habits with coffee, such as adding sugar, creamer, syrups, or drinking a pot a day, you need to make downsizing your coffee consumption a short-term goal. Caffeine is the number one drug in the world that people get addicted to. If you find yourself needing or simply wanting more than a cup in the morning, then you are officially addicted and you're going to have to go through the process of overcoming your addiction. This can be an uncomfortable process involving a few massive headaches from caffeine withdrawals. Now that you understand how the body works, don't justify "needing" coffee to make your headache go away. You're simply feeding your addiction. Allow your body to detox in whatever form your body needs, and embrace the uncomfortableness (headaches, cramps, digestive issues, etc.). You're the one that allowed your body to become so toxic and reliant on the drug. Knowingly or not, you got yourself addicted to coffee so take ownership. Remember, your health is your responsibility.

A last note on coffee: consuming coffee will suppress your appetite, so many people will drink it throughout the day and not eat anything because they're not hungry. This is not a good long-term strategy. Coffee is not nutrient dense, and you need to fuel your body appropriately. Don't wait until you're hungry to eat or you will overeat. Don't wait until your thirsty to drink; by that point your body is dehydrated. Be proactive with your food choices, and create daily rituals where you don't need to think about when and what you should be eating.

Lastly, think about what you can do to better maximize your time before you start the rest of your day. For example:

- If you drive to work or take the kids to school, give yourself plenty of extra time to arrive where you need to be. How can you arrive early so you can take your time parking, walking, and enjoying a slow and easy pace to wherever you're headed?

- If you have a commute to work, strengthen your mind by listening to podcasts or personal development audios rather than numbing your brain with talk radio or the same ten songs that are repeatedly on the radio. What would you enjoy learning? Find a podcast or audio program from the library that will help you fill your brain with good, positive energy.

- If you're a stay-at-home parent, listen to these same podcasts or audio programs when your kids are napping or while you're doing chores around the house. Just because you're staying home with your kids (which is the most important job of all) doesn't mean you have to stop learning. Plus, think about the example you're setting for your kids!

Fidelity Hour – How to Become Emotionally Connected to Your Loved Ones

Be sure to express your love as many ways as possible to your nearest and dearest before you take off in the morning. Whether it be your partner, children, or pets, make time for the most valuable people in your life by expressing love out loud, on paper, in hugs and kisses, and any other way you know how. Make your love palpable so you can all carry that affection with you for the rest of the day.

Marital fidelity is strengthened when you affirm your spouse, listen to your spouse, and seek to meet his or her needs – mentally, emotionally, and physically. Your relationship is also strengthened when you set healthy boundaries for your media consumption and for your relationships outside of the home.

Marital fidelity is weakened when you devalue your spouse, minimize the time you have with your spouse, and focus on meeting your own needs. That bond is also weakened when you fantasize about someone other than your spouse meeting your deepest needs and desires.

Turn the television off, put the phones away, get creative, and be spontaneous. If you're struggling to figure out where to begin, introduce the idea of picking a book to read through and discuss together. There are a ton of life-changing relationship books out there. Three of my personal favorites that have really impacted my love relationship are *The 5 Love Languages* by Gary Chapman, *His Needs Her Needs* by Willard F. Harley, and *Love Busters* also written by Willard F. Harley.

The Five Love Languages is what we gift every single couple when we are invited to their wedding. The book goes on to explain that there are five love languages and that everyone has one or two of them that tends to keep their love-tanks full. The five love languages include Acts of Service, Gifts, Quality of Time, Touch, and Words of Affirmation. Your spouse's love language is going to determine how you're going to best devote your time and energy to ensure you meet his or her needs and keep her feeling loved.

For instance, my wife's love languages are Words of Affirmation and Quality of Time. Simply put, she wants to experience present, conscious time with me, have quality conversations where we connect at a deep level, and spend time together where we're not on the clock or routinely being interrupted by kids, work, or social media. What "quality time" does not mean is simply talking about anything and everything (business, kids, sports, etc.) or spending time together while sitting on the couch watching television.

The fact that my wife likes Words of Affirmation and Quality of Time also means that the other three love languages are not going to have the same effect on her. She may enjoy them and appreciate them sporadically, but those other languages are not going to keep her feeling loved and appreciated. For instance, bringing home my wife flower (Gifts) is not going to have as much an impact on her feeling loved as if I were to acknowledge her for something good that she did that day and appreciate her for being a supportive mother to our kids and a wonderful wife to me. Another example is taking the trash out or drying the dishes (Acts of Service). Many times, these acts of service will go unnoticed when that love language doesn't fill the love-tank. My wife and I are extremely guilty of this. Because Acts of Service is not a top love language for either of us, we often take for granted the things we do around the house and for our family as if they're expected and simply part of our role as parents, homeowners, spouses, etc.

Now, of course, my wife's love languages may not be the same as your significant other's love languages. Your queen or king may enjoy spending time cuddling on the couch together or reading together or watching your favorite show together or going for a walk together. The key word is "together." It is important that you understand the five love languages, discover your spouse's love language, and learn to speak his or her love language. Doing so will equip you to better meet your spouse's need for love. Accomplishing this will take focused energy and making your relationship a priority.

Similar to the Power Hour, developing a short affirmation that you can use to jazz yourself up and refocus so that you are able to give all of your attention to your significant other is a wonderful strategy. Let's face it, after a long day, it's common to be drained and exhausted. You've given yourself and everyone else in your daily life your full attention, and now it's time to give your other half what he or she deserves. Make that time all about her, and strive to strengthen your relationship to a much deeper level and grow together.

Below is my "Fidelity Hour Affirmation" that I use to refocus myself after putting the kids to bed and before I spend time with my wife:

"Tonight is going to be a Phenomenal Night!

I am the Master of My Thoughts! I Determine how I Feel!!!"

[I close my eyes and take three deep breaths and I smile and feel it throughout my body.]

"Tonight, I will absolutely devote myself to Amanda.

I am Selfless.

I am open and honest.

Nothing matters at this moment other than Amanda.

I am curious about her feelings and her thoughts.

She deserves my full attention, and I will give it to her.

I will treat her like a queen.

Tonight, we will go to bed HAPPY and in LOVE!

It is my responsibility that Amanda feels safe and secure!

I will help her fall asleep because I want to."

Similar to how this book focuses on your health journey and the Six-Step Sequence to Extraordinary Health, you can take a very similar approach to your relationships. Change your mindset and make your significant other your number one priority, regardless of all the distractions and stressors that are keeping you busy. Come up with some relationship goals – first by yourself and eventually together with your partner. Create a game plan that is going to allow you and your spouse to have fun together, grow together, and ultimately keep each other's love-tanks full. Do not wait until either of your love-tanks are bone dry to try to address your relationship.

Lastly, celebrate the small victories and schedule fun and date nights with your significant other. I am no relationship expert; however, I cannot stress how important this is to your health and the quality of your life to strengthen your relationship with your partner.

Application Exercise #10

Now it's your turn. Take some time and write down what you'd like to include and do for your Power Hour, Fitness Hour, Morning Ritual, and Fidelity Hour. If you can't think of what to do, then use my personal examples above to get you started. The important part is write down your ideas now and start your rituals today or tomorrow. Over time, you'll figure out what works best for you.

For now, jot down some ideas... (You can download the "Transformational Rituals" and "Stop Doing List" worksheets at InspiredToBeHealthy.com)

During my Power Hour, I want to: _____

_____

_____

During my Fitness Hour, I want to: _____

_____

_____

During my Morning Ritual, I want to: _____

_____

_____

During our Fidelity Hour, I want to: _____

_____

_____

Stop Doing List – Everything I Do That Doesn't Push My Life Forward

Not only do you want to add the above rituals to your life, I also think taking some negative habits or rituals out of your life is just as important. Doing so will open your time up to more important rituals and help you live a more relaxed life.

What habits do you currently have that are not going to push you towards your health goals? Here are some common examples to help you get started:

I will stop hitting snooze and sleeping in.

I will stop checking my phone in the morning – email, social media, news, etc.

I will stop doing workouts that are boring and that do not push me to get better.

I will stop with impulse buys at the grocery store – snacks, sugar, wheat, dairy, etc.

I will stop listening to the radio on my car rides and instead put time and energy into sharpening my mindset.

I will stop wasting valuable time watching the news.

I will stop associating with negative people.

I will stop settling for the status quo.

Now, create your personal "Stop Doing" list. Feel free to use the examples above or create your own. Like your daily rituals, you will continually add to or tweak this list over time. Remember, the more things that don't move you forward toward your goals that you can stop doing, the more mentally, emotionally, and physically healthy actions, habits, and rituals you can add to your life to help you reach your goals.

I will stop. . . _____

I will stop. . . _____

I will stop. . . _____

I will stop. . . _____

I will stop. . . _____

I will stop. . . _____

I will stop. . . _____

Mentoring Moment

Game Changer: Commit to completing the Application Exercise and start your rituals as soon as possible. Then, continue to fine tune your rituals until you are exceeding your health goals as well as all other goals you have in your life.

Own It: To get the most out of this chapter, take the principles that you learned and teach them to someone else. As you begin to live out your daily rituals, you will learn what works and what doesn't, what is efficient and effective and what isn't. Once you can live out your daily rituals, take the time to share your personal rituals with others while teaching them the benefits. This will give you the opportunity to be a teacher and inspire others to be better!

15
Your Health
Your Responsibility

"Your health is your choice. Your health is your
responsibility; it's not anyone else's: It's not your
medical doctor's, not your health insurance company,
not your significant others, and it's certainly not
my responsibility. Your health is your responsibility."
Dr. Cotey Jordan

I have overcome chronic conditions, and I am now functioning to the best of my ability. I'm functioning better than I
have in my entire life. I am not telling you this to impress you. I
am telling you this to inspire you to do the same.

There is hope. You can do this. The healthy lifestyle I've created
was not because of my education; I totally wasted that. My
health didn't come as a result of my connections; I destroyed
them all. And I'm healthy not because I was lucky; I have never
been lucky at anything. I also didn't take some magic pill or
complete some get-healthy-quick program. Neither of these
"magic bullets" exist. The lifestyle I've created has helped me
overcome chronic illness and live an ultra-healthy life. The lifestyle you create can do the same for you.

You now know what millions of Americans don't. You know that health is not about symptoms; health is about removing any interference, so your body can function optimally. You know that health isn't someone else's responsibility – be it your doctor's, your health insurance company's, your spouse's. Health is your responsibility. And you now know how to take advantage of these facts using the Six Steps I've laid out for you here in this book to live an ultra-healthy lifestyle.

There are only a few more things left to do before we end our time together.

First, on the following pages, you'll find my personal strategies to stay ultra-healthy. I've included several lists in one place as well as a few smoothie recipes, so you can refer back to this book when you need help or to review what we've discussed.

Second, I suggest keeping this book in your possession and reviewing it until you learn how to appropriately use the Six-Step Sequence to an Extraordinary Life and the Core Four foundational principles of health, and you set up your daily rituals. Nothing happens without action. Please don't lay this book down and move on to another book or project. Fill out the Application Exercises, and start creating better habits and rituals for yourself.

For your convenience, I've compiled the Application Exercises and made them available for download as PDF's. You can download these resources at InspiredToBeHealthy.com.

Last, once you start having success, help others to do the same by getting them a copy of this book. Listen, if you care about someone in your life, then buying him a book (a resource that has over a decade of my experience and can shortcut his efforts) is a thoughtful gesture that he'll thank you for.

Remember, health is a journey and not a destination. As you reach your three-month and twelve-month goals, please reach out and make me one of the first people you celebrate with.

Your friend,

Dr. Cotey Jordan

My Personal Strategies to Stay Ultra-Healthy

My rituals are who I am. On the following pages, you'll see my personal strategies that have helped me become and stay ultra-healthy. Please feel free to adopt or modify any and all of these strategies to invest in your greatest asset – your health!

And if you're not familiar with one of the strategies, please understand that you may need to do some research to find out what some of these things are. You're here to grow and take responsibility for your health, so I have full confidence in you.

My Daily Rituals

1. Power Hour

2. Fitness Hour

3. Morning Ritual

4. Meal Plan / Food Prep

5. Fidelity Hour

6. Keep cell phone out of bedroom

What are your current daily rituals?

What do they need to be to reach your 30 year goals?

My Weekly Rituals

1. Meal Planning – Grocery shopping with purpose

2. Food Prep – Cooking with intention

3. Specific Chiropractic adjustments on a regular basis

4. Infrared sauna 3x week

5. Load Supplement trays for the week

6. Date night with my wife

7. Scheduled time with my kids

What are your current weekly rituals?

What do they need to be to reach your 30 year goals?

My Monthly Rituals

1. Modify fitness routine

2. Achieve then advance my goals

3. Update "Stop Doing" List

4. Read minimum of one book each month (personal growth)

5. Date night with one of my daughters

6. Reflect on Who I Am and Who I Am Becoming (Intellectual, emotional, character, spiritual)

What are your current monthly rituals?

What do they need to be to reach your 30 year goals?

My Health Cabinet

Ditch the Medicine Cabinet already!

1. Coconut Oil

2. Standard Process Supplements

3. Liquid Herbs

4. Essential Oils

5. Ice Packs

6. Epson Salt

7. Garlic / Onion

8. Apple Cider Vinegar

9. Homeopathy

What is in your health cabinet?

My Top 10
Health Investments

1. Lifetime Family Wellness Chiropractic Care

2. Full House Water Purification System

3. Consultation with a Whole Food Supplement Expert

4. Food Sensitivity Testing

5. Functional Neurology

6. Infrared Sauna

7. Diffusers – Essential Oils

8. Coach for every aspect of life (health coach, fitness coach, relationship coach, financial coach, business coach, etc.)

9. Industrial Blender for Smoothies (I personally use a BlendTec)

10. Home Gym or Gym Membership

What health investments are you currently making?

My Must-Use Devices

1. PEMF Mats

2. HBOT - Oxygen Concentrator

3. Cervical Traction Unit

4. Infrared Sauna

5. Spinal Hygiene

6. Industrial Blender - Blendtec

My TOP TEN Rituals
to Live Super Healthy

1. Get adjusted on a regular basis

2. Hydrate – Drink at least half your body weight in ounces each day

3. Take it or Eat it – Daily Supplements / Smoothies

4. Daily Workout + Protein Shake

5. Coconut Oil

6. Sugar/Wheat/Dairy Free

7. Spinal Hygiene

8. Stress Management

9. Food Planning / Meal Prep

10. Buy organic, non-GMO, whole foods

Favorite, Go-To Smoothies

(You can download videos of these favorite smoothie recipes being made at InspiredToBeHealthy.com)

Morning Zinger!

¼ apple

¼ pear

½ inch of ginger

Splash of lemon juice

Splash of lime juice

2 large handfuls of spinach

Water

Handful of ice cubes to make it cold

NOTE: This smoothie is mostly spinach and you can play with how much water you add depending on how liquid or thick you would like it. The flavor is good and the health benefits are even better! You can also play with the amount of ginger you add, the more you add the more zing there is. Typically, this makes a 32 oz. smoothie that I put into a mason jar and drink throughout the morning. Combine this smoothie with a veggie bowl, and you've set yourself up for a successful real food morning and afternoon!

Chocolate Protein Bliss!

[64 oz. yield]

1 Frozen Avocado

1 Heaping Spoon Cacao Powder

Spinach – two packed handfuls

2 servings Standard Process Complete Chocolate / Chocolate Bone Broth Powder

2-3 Cups Water / Coconut Milk

Ice – 2 to 3 handfuls

Need it sweeter? Optional add ins include:

- ½ Frozen Banana
- Tbsp Maple Syrup
- 4-8 Frozen Cherries

Peanut Butter Protein Bliss!

[64 oz. yield]

1 Frozen Avocado

1 Heaping Spoon Cacao Powder

Spinach – two packed handfuls

2 servings Standard Process Whey Pro (Protein Powder)

Peanut Butter – flavor to liking (4-6 Tbsp.)

2-3 Cups Water / Coconut Milk

Ice – 2 to 3 handfuls

Need it sweeter? Try adding in a half a banana or a little maple syrup.

*I also add a whole food product (Standard Process Complete) to my smoothies for added nutritional value.

May this book bring you love and joy for your entire existence.
That is my intention for you, and for the world.

To learn more about Dr. Cotey or have him speak at your event
please visit WellnessSpeakerUSA.com.

Made in the USA
Middletown, DE
10 November 2024

64014738R00133